T0231507

CLINICAL PROTOCOLS
in
LABOUR

CLINICAL PROTOCOLS
in
LABOUR

MICHAEL S. MARSH, MD, MRCOG
Senior Lecturer/Consultant in Obstetrics,
King's College Hospital, London, UK

JANET M. RENNIE, MA, MD, FRCP, FRCPCH, DCH
Consultant and Senior Lecturer in Neonatal Medicine,
King's College Hospital, London, UK

PHILLIPA A. GROVES, MBBS, DRCOG, FRCA
Consultant Anaesthetist,
King's College Hospital, London, UK

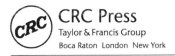
CRC Press
Taylor & Francis Group
Boca Raton London New York

CRC Press is an imprint of the
Taylor & Francis Group, an **informa** business

Published in the USA by
The Parthenon Publishing Group
345 Park Avenue South, 10th Floor
New York
New York 10010, USA

Published in the UK and Europe by
The Parthenon Publishing Group
23–25 Blades Court
Deodar Road, London
SW15 2NU, UK

Library of Congress Cataloging-in-Publication Data
Marsh, M. S. (Michael S.)
    Clinical protocols in labour / M.S. Marsh, J. Rennie, P. Groves.
        p. ; cm.
    Includes bibliographical references and index.
    ISBN 1-84214-085-X (pbk : alk paper)
    1. Labor (Obstetrics)--Complications. 2. Pregnancy--Complications. I. Rennie, Janet
M. II Groves, P. III. King's College (London, England) Hospital IV. Title
    [DNLM: 1. Labor Complications. 2. Delivery. 3. Pregnancy Complications--prevention
& control. WQ 330 M366c 2001]
    RG651 M345 2001
    618.5--dc21

                                                                    2001050060

British Library Cataloguing-in-Publication Data
Marsh, M. S. (Michael S.)
    Clinical protocols in labour
    1.Obstetrics - Practice
    I.Title II.Rennie, Janet M. III.Groves, P.
    618.2

    ISBN 184214085X

Typeset by H&H Graphics, Blackburn, UK

Contents

Introduction

The purpose of this book is to provide a useful guide to practice for midwives and doctors working on the labour ward. The aim is to outline the consensus of opinion that exists regarding the way in which various situations that may be encountered in labour are usually managed at King's College Hospital. Any plan of management should be discussed with the woman and her partner at all stages of labour.

Although using the King's College Hospital as a template, all techniques and recommendations herein are appropriate and relevant to the management of labour in other institutions. While the exact details of the King's protocols may vary from those from other hospitals, all information is designed to be applicable to the effective perinatal management of women and their babies.

Normally, care would be expected to follow a similar pattern to that outlined, but it is expected that on occasions individual circumstances will necessitate an alternative approach. When such a situation arises this should be discussed with the consultant and senior specialist registrar on call.

Some topics have been omitted where it was agreed that it was not possible to identify a general policy due to the high number of variables that could influence decision making – the management of a woman who has had two previous Caesarean sections being an obvious example. When such a situation arises the specialist registrar on call should always see the woman and then discuss the management plan with the on-call consultant.

Women who have high risk factors identified in the antenatal period should already have a plan for labour identified within their notes. The on-call obstetric specialist registrar should always be informed when such a woman is admitted in order that the care plan can be discussed again.

Labour ward protocols and guidelines should advance as new knowledge is gained in the field. A large well-conducted and widely disseminated study of a controversial area of obstetrics may change practice quite rapidly. The present protocol reflects the current practice at King's College Hospital, but this is very likely to change. For this reason, future editions are planned. The present edition takes into account recent guidelines from the National Institute for Clinical Excellence and the Royal College of Obstetrics and Gynaecology covering fetal monitoring in labour and induction of labour.

Acknowledgements

The present protocol is the result of a collaboration between many obstetricians, paediatricians, physicians and midwives at King's College Hospital over a number of years.

Special thanks should go to those listed below who have made substantial contributions to the protocol, to all other attendees of the Maternity Protocol Group and to other members of the department who have made important and helpful suggestions.

Midwives:	Cathy Warwick
	Verena Wallace
	Winsome Okeke
	Katie Yiannouzis
	Jill Demilew
	Becky Reid
	Jean Yearwood
Paediatricians	Anne Greenough
	Sean Devane
	Simon Hannam
Obstetricians	Donald Gibb
	Maggie Blott
	John Parsons
	Tony Davies
	Davor Jurkovic
	Lut Geerts
	Christoph Lees
Physicians	Adrian Stern
	Adrian Stephens
	Alex Mijovic

1

The approach to care

King's Healthcare provides maternity care to 4200 women a year. The women will be from a variety of social, ethnic and cultural backgrounds, so the circumstances of each individual will be unique. Some women will enter labour confident, happy and optimistic, others will be unsure, insecure and possibly frightened. Many will feel a combination of emotions depending on previous experience, knowledge and how labour progresses.

The challenge for the labour ward team is to create an environment that is supportive to the woman and her partner and makes them feel that their special circumstances and wishes are respected by those providing their care. It is important to remember that what may be routine and commonplace for staff may be strange and highly significant for the woman and her partner. It is essential that a team approach is fostered and that all matters relevant to the woman's care are documented to ensure that a cohesive and supportive approach is achieved.

It is essential that the woman's right to privacy is maintained and that unnecessary interruptions are avoided once the woman is in established labour. If it is necessary for a member of staff to enter a delivery room he/she should always knock on the door and await a reply before entering. On entering the room it is essential that he/she introduces him/herself to the woman and her partner and explains the reason for this involvement.

Women are actively encouraged to have a companion with them while they are on the labour ward. Some women may wish to have more than one person with them and normally this does not cause any problems. A request by a woman for a young child to attend the birth does present a particular challenge, but would not normally be refused provided the labour is straightforward and the child is well supported.

The importance of ascertaining the woman's wishes and ensuring that she is involved in discussions regarding her care cannot be over-emphasized. When a woman has a birth plan, its content should be discussed with her and her partner as appropriate in the later stages of the antenatal period. It is usually easy to agree on most of the points that are commonly raised. For example, an opt-out of routine syntocinon in the third stage for a low-risk pregnancy does not pose any problem. On the other hand, a twin pregnancy and a request for minimal intervention may cause difficulty. Such issues should be discussed with more senior members of staff. The birth plan should be signed and dated by a member of staff indicating that appropriate discussion has taken place. On admission to the labour ward, the existence of the birth plan must be acknowledged and its content reviewed again. Flexibility to the particular needs of the individual birth plan is a basic element of our care. Every woman should have the opportunity to discuss her plans for labour, and when this has occurred this should be recorded in the notes.

Most women giving birth at King's College Hospital will deliver normally. For those women whose labours veer from an anticipated pathway, staff caring for them should have an overall strategy for the labour, keeping the 'birth plan' in mind. Appropriate options can be considered to ensure the labour continues towards the best outcome possible.

RECORD KEEPING

In the records of pregnancy, birth and the postpartum period, salient clinical findings take precedence. The woman's record . . . 'should provide clear evidence of the care planned, the decisions made, the care delivered and the information shared . . .'[1]. This means that, for example, the reason for change of place of birth and how/why this decision was made, and by whom, should be recorded.

Colleagues consulted for advice or a second opinion should record their findings and, if required, the plan of action for pregnancy, labour and the puerperium in the woman's records. Any salient points should be transferred to the partogram and neonatal records as appropriate. Times of transfer and discharge should also be recorded, while dates and names should be written legibly on cardiotocography (CTG) traces. The name of the person on whom the CTG was performed, the date on which it was carried out and the point on the CTG when procedures, such as vaginal examinations, occurred should also be clearly indicated.

Guidelines for record keeping are as follows:

1. All entries must be legible and indelible, in permanent black ink. Any alterations should be crossed out using a single line.

2. Dates and times of entries must be clear. Entries must be written immediately after any patient contact.

3. Entries must be in chronological order and signed. Name, designation and bleep number must be printed under signature.

4. Every page must have the patient's name and hospital number.

5. Only use well recognised and relevant abbreviations and symbols.

6. Ensure allergies and specific instructions are clearly identified on front cover of notes.

7. There must be no unnecessary personal or subjective comments about the patient and/or family. Never use exclamation marks.

8. Details of verbal instructions or information given to the patient must be recorded.

9. All reports and results must be seen, evaluated and initialled by the responsible clinician before they are filed.

10. There should be regular progress notes throughout the patient's stay with at least a daily entry, and any unexpected events documented in full.

MANAGEMENT OF THE LABOUR WARD

Midwifery staff

Each day at King's College Hospital there are three shifts of midwives providing cover for the 24-h period, and on each shift one midwife is designated as being in charge overall. If any of the midwives working on a shift are having particular difficulties, they should discuss them with the midwife-in-charge. The midwife-in-charge should accompany the medical team when they undertake the hand-over round.

Some women will be cared for by practice midwives and community midwives. Women with uncomplicated pregnancies normally have their care provided totally by midwives. Midwives are expected, once they have been taught, to suture the perineum and to set up intravenous infusions.

The midwife should identify women with complicated pregnancies on admission. The specialist registrar should be informed of the women's arrival by the midwife and he/she should see the woman promptly. The specialist registrar is personally responsible for reviewing the case.

At King's College Hospital on most occasions one consultant, senior specialist registrar, junior specialist registrar and senior house officer (SHO) are designated for labour ward duties each day. There is at least one doctor present on the labour ward at all times, and SHOs operate on a shift system. The on-call consultant is available for teaching, training and advice and in the event of complications arising.

Medical staff

The role of the SHO is to assist, if requested, with the care of women with uncomplicated pregnancies, for example suturing the perineum. The SHOs are expected to work alongside the specialist registrar and midwives in order to observe and learn about the management of complicated and uncomplicated pregnancies. The SHO must discuss all cases with the specialist registrar.

DAILY WARD REVIEW

Every week-day there is a consultant-led labour ward review at 08:30 (or thereabouts) where the care of women with problems is reviewed. The primary purpose of this review is to ensure that all aspects of the woman's care are discussed with the team taking over so a consistent pattern of care is achieved. Women in normal labour do not need to be formally reviewed on the ward round, but these women must be asked if they wish to see the medical team at this time. The team taking over must attend this review promptly, as must the specialist registrar and SHO going off duty. The hand-over report will be given by the most appropriate person, normally the midwife providing care, the SHO or a medical or midwifery student. Ideally, the review should finish within 1–1.5 h. The ward round will continue on the intensive care unit as necessary. Intensive care patients may be reviewed by the team of the relevant consultant.

The review should be used as a learning opportunity for more junior staff and medical students, and they should be encouraged to participate in the presentation and discussion of case histories. It is important that this review does not interfere with the mother's privacy and discussion should take place outside the room. Women in normal labour need not be reviewed by medical staff unless the midwife caring for her feels it appropriate or the mother wishes it. Additional rounds by the senior specialist registrar, junior specialist registrar and SHO should take place at every 4–5 h during the day. The senior specialist registrar should always contact the consultant on call following the last round of the day.

STUDENTS

Midwifery, medical and nursing students are allocated to the labour ward and gain their experience working with the mothers, midwives and doctors. It is essential that all women are asked if they wish for student participation in their care. If a woman does not wish to have a student take part in her care this request should be respected and recorded. A delivery may be conducted by a student only if that student has helped to care for that woman for a significant time prior to the delivery.

STAFFING LEVELS

If at any time the midwife in charge and/or the specialist registrar on duty for the labour ward feels that the level of staffing is inconsistent with safe care they should contact the senior midwife in charge of the unit, the supervisor of midwives and the on-call consultants (see appendix 1)

REFERENCE

1. UKCC 1998. *Guidelines for records and record keeping.* London: UKCC, 1998

2

Domino/GPO and home deliveries

DOMINO DELIVERIES

Women booked for Domino deliveries will have had the majority of their antenatal care in the community and have been cared for by a community-based midwife often in conjunction with a General Practitioner Obstetrician (GPO). When a woman is in labour, she will either ring the labour ward or will telephone the 'on-call' midwife from the midwifery practice.

AREA COMMUNITY MIDWIVES

When the woman arrives at the hospital for the birth, one of the labour ward midwives will examine the woman. If labour is established, the labour ward midwife will contact the on-call area midwife.

PRACTICE MIDWIVES

In the antenatal period, women are advised to contact the on-call practice midwife by pager when in labour. The practice midwife will then decide whether to visit the woman at home or come to the hospital to meet the woman and care for her throughout labour.

In certain circumstances, labour ward midwives will have to provide cover for area or practice midwives. This will only happen if the on-call midwives are attending a home birth – the midwife on call has already been up for a long time and is not safe to remain on duty – or there is a shortage of midwives.

Midwifery care for induction of labour is negotiated on an ad hoc basis. Generally, the area midwives do not cover induction, and the midwifery practices provide labour ward care when the labour is well established. Women should be informed during their pregnancy that this may be the situation.

Following the delivery, the mother is transferred to the postnatal ward in the normal way and usually transferred home within 6–48 h. If the woman wishes to go home directly from the labour ward, this should be possible if this agreed by the care givers.

GUIDELINES FOR COMMUNITY MIDWIVES ON HOME BIRTHS

Background

The Changing Childbirth Report[1] focuses on three principles: choice, control and continuity. All women requesting a home birth should be supported in their choice. However, if a woman is thought to be at any risk during the pregnancy, she will be told of the risk and appropriate advice given. Midwives should adopt an holistic approach to care provision according to the physical, psychosocial, cultural, spiritual and educational needs of individual women and their families in the home environment.

Women residing within the immediate surrounding area will normally be cared for by the hospital's midwives and obstetricians. For those women living outside this area (which should be previously determined), a senior midwife or supervisor of midwives will assess a request for a home birth before a final decision is reached. Efficient and effective use of midwifery resources must be taken into account at all times.

Fragmentation of the service can result when midwives cross normal boundaries to deliver care. Although women from outside the area may be cared for during the antenatal and intrapartum periods, they will normally return to their local midwives for postnatal care.

Overview

It is fundamental that the mother takes part in all decisions made throughout the pregnancy, during labour and during the postnatal period. A flexible and supportive approach should be taken that involves midwives sharing their professional knowledge and expertise with individual mothers. This is in the belief that women need to be equipped with the appropriate information to assist them in identifying their own health needs.

TABLE 2-1. AIMS OF THE HOME BIRTH SERVICE

* To encourage and emphasize the importance of a healthy lifestyle and good nutrition during pregnancy
* To educate women in identifying their own health needs and to seek help if necessary
* To monitor the emotional and psychological changes during the antenatal, intrapartum and early postnatal periods
* To plan care with the mother while fostering a partnership in respect of her individual, cultural, psychosocial and educational needs
* To encourage the woman to attend parent education classes, especially if it is her first baby
* To actively promote and encourage breastfeeding amongst all mothers and to provide them with evidence to help them in making a decision
* To provide mothers with the appropriate level of support in their preferred choice of feeding
* To be supportive of the woman's chosen birth partner

Organization of antenatal care

Protocols need to be defined so that there is organized antenatal care at the general practitioner's surgery or other facility as appropriately arranged. Moreover, the woman should be familiar with the ways in which she can contact a midwife when she is in labour, if she has a problem or needs advice. This information is contained within her hand-held notes.

Organization – labour and the birth

In the UK, the *MIDIRS* (Midwives Information and Resource Service) leaflet on Informed Choice should be available to women to assist them in choosing their place of delivery (patients should always be informed of literature that can help in deciding their course). When a home birth is planned, appropriate back-up arrangements should be in place so that the woman knows whom to contact if her named midwife or her named team of midwives is not immediately available. All Community and Practice midwives must give the woman the number of the on-call pager and how to make contact when she is in labour. The labour ward telephone number should also be given to women, but she should be told that this only be called if she cannot get her midwife via her pager.

A midwife attending a home birth must always have a well-charged mobile telephone or access to a telephone. If the midwife assesses via telephone that the birth is not imminent and the woman can cope, the midwife should first go to the hospital to collect the home birth equipment and take it to the home. If there is no urgency, only one midwife needs to go to the woman's home regardless of the time of day or night, but the midwife in charge of the labour ward must always be notified whenever a home birth is underway should there be a need for transfer to hospital.

When the midwife arrives at the home to assess the progress of labour, if the woman is in early labour and would not benefit from the midwife staying in the home, the midwife may leave, but agree with the woman when to call again. The midwife should ensure the woman has all the necessary contact telephone numbers before she leaves. The midwife should also make contact if she does not hear from the woman within an agreed time.

When the midwife visits the woman for the first time in labour, a detailed history of the events is taken and full abdominal examination is performed to ascertain the frequency and duration of any contractions. An examination to determine whether the membranes are ruptured may be performed.

There should be adequate and regular recordings of the fetal heart rate, maternal vital signs (temperature, pulse and blood pressure) and labour progress. Clear documentation of all these features can be achieved by the use of the partogram, which would alert the midwife when a delay in progress of labour is apparent. Records should be timed and legibly signed[2,3].

A fetal Doppler ultrasound should be available to establish the presence of a fetal heartbeat. Any difficulty in hearing the fetal heart with the Doppler equipment should be reported to the senior specialist registrar on call and arrangements made for the mother's transfer to the labour ward after alerting the midwife in charge with the reasons for transfer[3].

The fetal heart should be listened to every 15–30 min in the first stage of labour and every 5 min (approximately) in the second stage. The heart should be listened to during and after a contraction for a minimum of 60 s. Special care should be taken to ensure that the 'fetal heart rate' is not the maternal pulse, particularly when there is maternal tachycardia.

The 2001 recommendations from the National Institute for Clinical Excellence (NICE) and the Royal College of Obstetricians and Gynaecologists (RCOG) on fetal monitoring in labour suggest that continuous electronic fetal monitoring (and therefore hospital delivery) be "offered and recommended" in the following circumstances: previous Caesarean section; pre-eclampsia; a pregnancy of longer than 42 weeks; rupture of membranes longer than 24 h; induced labour; diabetes; antepartum haemorrhage; other maternal medical disease; intrauterine growth retardation; prematurity; oligohydramnios; abnormal Doppler artery velocimetry; multiple pregnancy; meconium-stained liquor; and breech presentation. In cases where such factors are identified antenatally then the risks and benefits of home versus hospital and intermittent versus continuous electronic fetal monitoring (CEFM) should be discussed between the relevant consultant, the woman and her midwife. If identified for the first time in labour at home these issues should be discussed with the woman and documented clearly in the notes.

The evidence for the benefits of CEFM over intermittent monitoring is weaker for some categories than others, e.g. pregnancy of longer than 42 weeks, rupture of membranes of over 24 h and induction of labour with prostaglandins.

If the birth is anticipated to be imminent, the first midwife will call a second midwife to collect the equipment and will herself go directly to the home to assess the progress of labour.

Every midwife must have a disposable delivery pack in her car at all times when she is at work. Appropriate equipment for neonatal resuscitation and adequate training and annual updates in the use of bag and mask ventilation are required of all midwives undertaking a home delivery[3]. Every midwife must be able to detect any deviation from the normal in either the mother or the baby and must make prompt referral to the consultant obstetrician/neonatologist or senior specialist registrar.

Under normal circumstances and towards the end of the first stage of labour, the first midwife will call the second midwife as her assistant. The woman and her birth partner should have previously been told that a second midwife would be in attendance at the birth.

After the woman and her baby are both made comfortable and the documentation of the birth is completed, the midwife will leave the home and take all equipment back to the hospital for cleaning and storage or disposal.

Arrangements must be made for the baby to have a neonatal examination within 72 h of the birth. The midwife should have made appropriate arrangements for the neonatal examination in the antenatal period. This will entail either the woman's primary care physician coming to examine the baby or the woman taking the baby to the neonatal ward for examination. To avoid an unnecessary wait, it is advisable for the midwife to make an appointment with the neonatal ward prior to the woman being sent to the hospital.

The hand-written Notification of Birth must be taken back to the community office at the hospital as soon as possible after the birth – ideally when the equipment is returned.

Health and safety

Normally, one midwife will go alone in the first instance to a home birth and the second midwife will be called towards the end of the first stage of labour. If there is a feeling of insecurity in isolated or unusual addresses, at night, or if it is strongly felt that two midwives should go out together, this must be discussed with the supervisor of midwives. A documented plan of action should then be agreed. Efficient and effective use of midwifery resources and the safety of midwives must be taken into account at all times.

The midwife must at all times telephone the midwife in charge of the labour ward informing her that she is going out to a home birth alone and agree that she will call again on arrival. An alarm must then be raised within an agreed time if there is no contact. Personal alarms are advisable to all midwives in the community, while all midwives attending a homebirth should take their team's mobile phone and on-call pager with them.Women must be informed never to leave urgent messages on the answering machine in the community midwives office.

TABLE 2-2. TRAINING REQUIREMENTS OF MIDWIVES IN-CHARGE OF HOME BIRTHS

Midwives should be able to:
- suture the perineum
- insert an intravenous cannula
- undertake bag and mask resuscitation of the baby
- know the emergency 'drill' for shoulder dystocia
- give emergency care in a catastrophic postpartum haemorrhage
- undertake an adult resuscitation and
- manage a newly diagnosed breech

TABLE 2-3. STANDARDS FOR MIDWIVES UNDERTAKING HOME BIRTHS

Standard	Monitoring method
All women should be provided with realistic and evidence-based information regarding their choice and place of birth. Trust in the midwife is of paramount importance to the woman and her partner	Woman's notes
To undertake 90% of the initial history taking (bookings) for women requesting this service	Woman's notes and EuroKing
To provide 90% of the antenatal care for low-risk pregnant women in the GP's surgery, their homes or at the hospital by a familiar midwife. This is to establish continuity of care and carer	Woman's notes
To ensure that all women booked for homebirths meet all midwives within the team by the time they are 37 completed weeks' gestation, or before labour is established if the decision for a home birth was made late into the pregnancy	Woman's notes
To support women in drawing up a birth plan in which they can outline their hopes and wishes for the birth	Woman's notes
All midwives should be confident or competent in all aspects of maternity care before taking charge of a home birth. If the experience is in any way compromised, the midwife and senior midwife alike must collaborate to ensure that this is in place	Performance appraisal
To refer and inform an obstetrician or senior midwife/supervisor of midwives of all women whom a midwife believes that there are reasons why a home birth should not be recommended, i.e. if the woman insists	Woman's notes
All records must be maintained and with a legible signature	Woman's notes
The community senior midwife should be informed of all potential home births	Computer records
The Notification of Birth must be handed in to the community office within 24 h of delivery	Community records

MECONIUM-STAINED LIQUOR DURING HOME BIRTHS

When meconium-stained liquor occurs during home births, the following factors must be considered before a decision is reached as to whether it is necessary to transfer the woman into hospital for delivery:

- The clinical situation should be reviewed for risk factors such as a smaller-than expected baby

- Although it has been shown to be difficult to classify meconium staining accurately[4], in women with light meconium staining of the liquor, the risk of meconium aspiration syndrome is low (0.3–1%), as is the risk of intrapartum hypoxia[5]. Women who are thought to have light meconium staining should be informed that the department advises delivery in hospital with a paediatrician present and that the NICE/ RCOG guidelines advise CEFM. Discussions regarding home versus hospital delivery should be documented in detail in the notes

The midwife must ensure that an ambulance is called and the woman transported to the labour ward.

All midwives undertaking home births are reminded that they must ensure that their neonatal resuscitation skills are updated regularly. Updating should be at least annual.

Equipment for resuscitation in the home should be checked daily by the on-call midwife as part of the routine check of homebirth equipment, in case repairs or replacements are necessary, and it should always be checked immediately before a home birth and after each delivery.

EMERGENCIES AT A HOMEBIRTH

Emergencies are rare during home births, and all the eventualities cannot be covered in home birth guidelines, but the principles are that if an emergency occurs, the midwife should contact a senior obstetrician (senior specialist registrar or consultant on call) at the hospital for advice and guidance, call a paramedic ambulance and keep the parents informed.

The procedures for obstetric emergencies are described elsewhere in these guidelines.

Many hospitals do not have an obstetric or paediatric 'flying squad'. If medical advice is needed, the midwife should always contact the senior specialist registrar/consultant on call in either obstetrics or neonatology directly for advice and guidance.

If labour is precipitate and is likely to occur as an unplanned delivery at home, or if it is anticipated that the baby will need resuscitation and/or transfer after delivery, an ambulance should be called and the neonatology department should be informed prior to delivery.

For a neonate requiring resuscitation following delivery, neonatal resuscitation guidelines should be followed and there should be no attempt to intubate unless a person with these skills is present, since it is too easy to do harm to the baby if this is not a procedure that is practised regularly. The 'bag and mask' technique should be performed to keep the baby alive until the paramedic arrives and the baby is admitted to hospital. Babies with a heart rate below 100 beats/min need chest compression.

The principle for an emergency at a home birth is that the midwife carries on providing the clinical care, following guidance for obstetric emergencies and his/her assistant does the following:

- calls the ambulance and states paramedic needed
- phones the labour ward and talks to an obstetrician (senior specialist registrar/consultant on call), asking them to tell the midwife in charge of the neonate's imminent arrival and
- writes contemporaneous notes

If any woman needs transfer from a home birth to the labour ward for any reasons other than purely for analgesia, the senior specialist registrar in obstetrics on call must be informed.

GUIDELINES FOR MANAGEMENT OF EMERGENCIES AT A HOME BIRTH

For the management of antepartum haemorrhage, shoulder dystocia, postpartum haemorrhage, definite retained placenta and cord prolapse at a home birth, see tables 2.4–2.8.

TABLE 2-4. GUIDELINES FOR MANAGEMENT OF ANTEPARTUM HAEMORRHAGE AT A HOME BIRTH

Midwife	Assistant
Insert intravenous (IV) cannula	Call the ambulance and state paramedic needed
Put up IV normal saline 1 l	Phone labour ward and talk to obstetrician (specialist registrar/senior specialist registrar/consultant); ask them to tell midwife in charge of your imminent arrival
Monitor the baby's heart rate Monitor the mother's vital signs	Write contemporaneous notes

TABLE 2-5. GUIDELINES FOR MANAGEMENT OF SHOULDER DYSTOCIA AT A HOME BIRTH

Midwife	Assistant
Follow guidelines for shoulder dystocia below	Call the ambulance and state paramedic needed
	If possible, talk through procedure with obstetrician (senior specialist registrar/ consultant on call) and relay to midwife
	Prepare to resuscitate baby

TABLE 2-6. GUIDELINES FOR MANAGEMENT OF POSTPARTUM HAEMORRHAGE AT A HOME BIRTH (ongoing loss of > 1 l) (see also chapter 26)

Midwife	Assistant
If the third stage of labour was physiological, give intra muscular (IM) syntometrine 1 ampoule	
Insert intravenous (IV) cannula	Call the ambulance and state paramedic needed

Continued

TABLE 2-6. (continued)

Put up IV normal saline 1 l with 100 units syntocinon and plasma expander, e.g. Haemaccel	Phone labour ward and talk to obstetrician (specialist registrar/senior specialist registrar/consultant on call); ask them to tell midwife in charge of your imminent arrival
Monitor mother's vital signs at least every 15 min	Write contemporaneous notes

TABLE 2-7. GUIDELINES FOR MANAGEMENT OF DEFINITE RETAINED PLACENTA AT A HOME BIRTH

Midwife	Assistant
Insert intravenous (IV) cannula	Call the ambulance and state paramedic
Monitor the mother's vital signs	Phone labour ward and talk to obstetrician
If bleeding is more than 1 l and ongoing, put up IV normal saline 1 l with 100 units syntocinon and plasma expander, e.g. Haemaccel	(specialist registrar/senior specialist registrar/consultant); ask them to tell midwife in charge of your imminent arrival
Observe blood loss carefully	Write contemporaneous notes
Insert indwelling catheter	

TABLE 2-8. GUIDELINES FOR MANAGEMENT OF CORD PROLAPSE AT A HOME BIRTH

Midwife	Assistant
Replace cord in vagina	Call the ambulance and state paramedic
Position mother with pelvis elevated	Phone labour ward and talk to obstetrician (specialist registrar/senior specialist registrar/consultant); ask them to tell midwife in charge of your imminent arrival
Move presenting part upwards with a hand in the vagina. This hand should be kept in place thoughout transfer until delivery	Write contemporaneous notes

Newly-diagnosed breech at a home birth (see also Chapter 21)
It is important to decide whether to continue care at home or in hospital. If delivery is not imminent the woman should be transferrred.

If decision is for transfer to hospital, call an ambulance and state urgent transfer and why – you will accompany woman in the ambulance. Take the delivery pack, oxytocics and neonatal resuscitation kit. Advise the ambulance crew to take you to the most appropriate hospital entrance for the time of day. Call the labour ward, ask to speak to the labour ward co-ordinator (sister in charge) and give her a summary of the admission.

If delivery appears to be imminent, get help (either telephone for help by oneself or ask the woman's partner to do so) and call a second midwife to come. Call an ambulance. It may be possible to revise your decision to stay at home if the second stage takes longer than anticipated. Request a paramedic for neonatal transfer in the event of the baby requiring continuing care in hospital, preparing equipment fully and anticipating the fact that resuscitation of the baby may be necessary. Telephone the labour ward to talk through delivery with competent clinician (specialist registrar/senior specialist registrar/consultant on call). Finally, ensure that the room in which the delivery is to take place is warm and/or prepare warm towels. It must also be remembered that contemporaneous notes should be written throughout.

The birth of a newly-diagnosed breech: general principles
Never pull or apply any traction, because this can cause mechanical problems (e.g. with the arms extending or the head not flexing effectively causing delayed delivery of the head). Never grasp the baby around the abdomen because this may cause trauma to the abdominal organs

Do not rush. Once the baby is born to the nape of the neck (hairline), gently support the baby to enable smooth delivery of the head. Be ready to resuscitate the baby should he/she need it.

Standing breech delivery
Until further studies of standing breech delivery are available, this position for delivery is not recommended and staff are advised not to use this method of breech delivery. Anecdotal reports suggest a high risk of fetal morbidity and mortality.

TABLE 2-9. REQUIRED EQUIPMENT AND DRUGS FOR HOME BIRTH

Equipment List	Drugs carried
Urine testing equipment	Lotions
Bottles and forms for blood tests	Analgesics
Needles and syringes	Laxatives
Lancets for dextrostix test etc.	Narcan
Stethoscope	Konakion (Intramuscular (IM) & oral)
Sonicaid and/or Pinard stethoscope	Obstetric cream/KY jelly
Sphygmomanometer	1% Lidocaine
Thermometer	Oxytoxics
Low-reading thermometer	
Three-way catheter	

Delivery Equipment
Disposable gloves/apron
Vaginal examination pack or equivalent bowl/receivers
Delivery pack or equivalent bowl/receivers/artery forceps
Suturing material, needles and instruments
Dissecting forceps
Needle holder
Scissors
Episiotomy scissors
Cord scissors
Cord clamps/ligatures
Baby resuscitation equipment including mucous extractor (double trap)
Adult resuscitation equipment
O_2
Entonox
Baby scales
Tape measure
Indwelling catheter and bag
Urethral catheters
Grey venflon × 4
Giving sets × 2

Intravenous (IV) fluids	1 × Hartmann's solution
	1 l N saline
	100 iu syntocinon
	2 units plasma substitute

REFERENCES

1. Cumberlege JF, and the Expert Maternity Group. Changing Childbirth. London: The Stationery Office, 1993
2. Clements RV. *Safe Practice in Obstetrics and Gynaecology.* Edinburgh: Churchill Livingstone, 1994:492
3. Fifth Annual Report of the Confidential Enquiry into Stillbirths and Deaths in Infancy. London: CESDI, 1996
4. van Heijst ML, van Roosmalen G, Keirse MJ. Classifying meconium-stained liquor: is it feasible? Birth 1995;22:191–5
5. Yong YP, Ho LY. A 3-year review of meconium aspiration syndrome. Singapore Med J 1997;38:205–8

BIBLIOGRAPHY

Croughan-Minihane MS, Pettiti DB, Giordis L, Golditch I. Morbidity among breech infants according to method of delivery. *Obstet Gynecol* 1990;75: 821–5

de Swiet M, ed. *Medical Disorders in Obstetric Practise,* 4th edn. Oxford, UK: Blackwell Science, 1995:683

Edmonds DK, ed. *Dewhurst's Textbook of Obstetrics and Gynaecology for Postgraduates,* 6th edn. Oxford, UK: Blackwell Science, 1999:622

James DK, *et al.* High Risk Pregnancy. London: WB Saunders, 1994:1318

Leung WC, Pun TC, Wong WM. Undiagnosed breech revisited. *Br J Obstet Gynaecol* 1999;106:638–41

Lindqvist A, Norden-Lindenberg S, Hanson U. Perinatal mortality and route of delivery in term breech presentations. *Br J Obstet Gynaecol* 1997;104: 1288–91

Nwosu EC, Walkinshaw S, Chia P, Manasse PR, Atlay RD. Undiagnosed breech. *Br J Obstet Gynaecol* 1993;100:531–5

The Use of Electronic Fetal Monitoring: the Use and Interpretation of Cardiotocography in Intrapartum Fetal Surveillance (Guideline no. 8). London: RCOG Press, 2001

3

Normal labour

DEFINITION OF LABOUR

Progressive dilatation of the uterine cervix in association with repetitive uterine contractions

DEFINITION OF THE ONSET OF LABOUR

Continued and regular uterine contractions and dilatation of the uterine cervix of 3 cm or more

ADMISSION CRITERIA

A woman will usually contact her practice midwife or telephone the labour ward for advice. If a woman gives a history of any of the following, she should be asked to come in:

- A contraction pattern that suggests that labour is established

- A history suggestive of rupture of the membranes (unless she can be assessed by the practice midwife in the clinic or at home)

- Vaginal bleeding

- Advised during the antenatal period to present early in labour

- A high-risk situation

Women who are having infrequent contractions may be advised to stay at home until one of the criteria listed above is achieved. If the woman seems worried or concerned, she should be advised to come to the labour ward for assessment.

FETAL ASSESSMENT UNIT REFERRALS

Women should be asked to attend the fetal assessment unit on the specified days and within the specified hours of opening if they fulfil the following criteria:

- A possibility of ruptured membranes at term
- Reduced fetal movements (< 10 per day)
- Pervaginal bleeding of less than 1 teaspoonful
- Unexplained mild abdominal pain

When advice is given to a woman as a result of a telephone enquiry, a note should be made in the book kept on the labour ward.

ADMISSION PROCEDURE

Each woman should be admitted by the midwife allocated to care for her. The antenatal files of patient history must be obtained from the antenatal clinic if possible, as these may contain important notes associated with medical problems and social circumstances. Any antenatal risk factors should be established from the woman and her notes, and if risk factors are present, the senior house officer (SHO) or specialist registrar should be asked to see the woman on admission.

The woman and her partner should be made welcome and the woman's companion made familiar with the environment, for example where to obtain refreshments and where the visitors' room and phone are located. They should also be informed of the way events are likely to proceed. This should be a two-way discussion and any special wishes/requests for labour that the woman may have should be noted. The woman's own plan for her birth should be taken into account.

The woman should know the name(s) of the midwife, student midwife and/or doctor (if appropriate) who are caring for her and should also be asked whether it is acceptable to her for medical or nursing students to be involved in her care. The result of this discussion should always be recorded in the woman's notes.

Checks should be made to ensure that a recent (within 16 weeks) normal (> 10 mg/dl) Hb result is available. If not, blood for full blood count testing should be taken.

An abdominal examination should be performed soon after the woman has been made comfortable.

Monitoring of fetal heart in low-risk women who are thought to be in labour, either by cardiotocography (CTG) or intermittent auscultation, should be commenced within 30 min of admission to the labour ward. An admission CTG need not be performed in women who have had a normal pregnancy, who have no risk factors and in whom the fetus is appropriately grown. It should not be considered a routine procedure in such low-risk women. There is some evidence that in such women an admission CTG increases the risk of operative delivery without fetal or maternal benefit[1]. The decision to perform an admission CTG should be discussed with the woman and her partner. If an admission CTG is performed it should continue until 2 accelerations (a rise of 15 bpm for 15 s above baseline rate) have been seen and the baseline variability (> 5 bpm) and baseline rate (110–160 bpm) confirmed as normal. If this is done when the fetus is active, it may be short. Otherwise, it may take 20 min or more. It is important to consider actively when to stop this trace and to inform medical staff promptly if it is abnormal.

If the CTG is normal, it may be repeated at 3–4 h intervals. It is not necessary for the mother to be lying down whilst the CTG is being performed. If the woman is in established labour, she may feel more comfortable standing, and it is normally possible to obtain a satisfactory trace in this way. Alternatively, she may wish to sit in a comfortable chair. Baseline observations should be taken soon after admission and a partogram commenced when the woman is in labour.

At the onset of labour, the resuscitaire and equipment for neonatal resuscitation in the room should be checked. If adequate equipment is not available, the midwife in charge of the labour ward should be informed.

INTERMITTENT AUSCULATION FOR MONITORING THE FETAL HEART IN LABOUR

The fetal heart should be listened to every 15–30 min in the first stage and every 5 min or around every contraction in the second stage. The heart should be listened to during and after a contraction for a minimum of 60 s. Special care should be taken to ensure that the fetal heart rate is not really the maternal pulse, in particular when there is maternal tachycardia. The 2001 National Institute for Clinical Excellence and Royal College of Obstetricians and Gynaecologists recommendations on fetal monitoring in labour[2] suggest that continuous electronic fetal monitoring be "offered and recommended" in the following circumstances:

- Previous Caesarean section
- Pre-eclampsia
- Pregnancy > 42 weeks
- Rupture of membranes > 24 h
- Induced labour
- Diabetes
- Antepartum haemorrhage
- Other maternal medical disease
- Intrauterine growth retardation
- Prematurity
- Oligohydramnios
- Abnormal Doppler artery velocimetry
- Multiple pregnancy
- Meconium stained liquor and
- Breech presentation

In cases where such factors are identified then the risks and benefits of intermittent versus continuous electrical fetal monitoring (CEFM) should be discussed between the obstetric staff, the woman and her midwife, and documented clearly in the notes.

The evidence for the benefit of CEFM over intermittent monitoring is weaker for some categories than others, e.g. pregnancy of longer than 42 weeks, rupture of membranes over 24 h previously and induction of labour with prostaglandins.

USE OF THE PARTOGRAM AND NORMOGRAM

The chief purpose of the partogram is to enable efficient and effective communication between professionals. The use of the partogram does not imply a dogmatic approach to the management of normal labour.

If a certain diagnosis of labour is difficult to make, the woman should have a short assessment period (1–2 h) on the labour ward. Recordings should then be made in the antenatal section of the clinical notes. If not in established labour, the woman may go home or to the ward if indicated (or if she so chooses).

A partogram should be commenced as soon as the onset of labour has been diagnosed, unless delivery is perceived to be imminent. Before labour is established, recordings should be made in the antenatal section of the clinical notes. Women at low risk who are not in established labour should not usually be managed on the labour ward.

According to its layout, any unusual features should be marked in the special features box of the partogram. The symphysis fundal height and clinical estimate of fetal weight or any other defined measurement should be entered in the space provided for this purpose.

It is essential that all the necessary observations are recorded clearly on the partogram. The situation should be fully explained to the woman and her partner and, with their consent, a plan of management must be made and clearly documented in the notes.

If the pregnancy is less than 36 weeks' gestation, the specialist registrar should be informed of the woman's admission and he/she should assess the woman. The neonatal unit, the woman and her partner should be involved in all discussions regarding how her care is to be managed, and the specialist paediatric registrar should also be informed.

CERVICAL DILATATION AS A GUIDE TO PROGRESS

Once the onset of labour is established, a partogram should be started and vaginal examination should be performed at least every 4 h. An abdominal palpation must be performed with every vaginal examination and documented in the notes. If the progress of cervical dilatation is 0.5 cm/h or less, referral to the medical staff is essential and a full discussion of further management needs to occur between the labouring woman, her attendants, her midwife and the obstetric specialist registrar.

It is usual under these circumstances for an artificial rupture of membranes (ARM) to be suggested followed by a vaginal examination after 2 h. If, after this time, the cervical dilatation has not changed, then an infusion of syntocinon may be commenced. A repeat vaginal examination should be performed if there has been a delay in starting syntocinon of over 1 h. ARM must be performed prior to commencing syntocinon.

Pre-labour rupture of membranes at term with engaged cephalic presentation

If the membranes have obviously ruptured (e.g. liquor is present at the vulva), but there is no history of contractions, in order to minimize the risk of infection, a vaginal speculum or examination need not be performed. If the diagnosis is uncertain, a speculum examination should be performed. If the diagnosis remains uncertain and the history is strongly suggestive of rupture of membranes (ROM), an ultrasound (US) scan may be arranged to assess liquor volume. However, it must be understood that a normal liquor volume on US does not exclude ROM. An US scan is not necessary if the diagnosis is clear.

A low vaginal swab should also be taken and sent for culture and sensitivity. The laboratory should be informed that the swab has been taken and arrangements should be made for this to be 'plated' as soon as possible. If the swab has been taken at night it will be plated first thing in the morning. If the diagnosis of ROM is uncertain, the woman should be asked to wear a pad and report any further leakage. If ROM is confirmed, under normal circumstances the woman should be transferred home or to the antenatal ward and the onset of labour awaited. In some instances though, especially if the woman is anxious, it may be more appropriate for her to be transferred to the antenatal ward overnight. The temperature should be taken every 6 h and the fetal heart monitored with a 20 min CTG or continuously for 10 min with a sonicaid every 24 h. If labour does not commence within 48–96 h, the risks of expectant management versus stimulation will need to be discussed.

If the pregnancy is less than 36 weeks' gestation, the specialist registrar should be informed of the woman's admission and he/she should assess the woman.

VAGINAL EXAMINATION

A vaginal examination should always be preceded by an abdominal examination. At vaginal examination, the following should be assessed: cervical dilatation, effacement and application, intactness of membranes, colour of liquor, fetal head position, station, moulding and caput. If an ARM is performed, the indication should be clearly written in the notes.

Ambulation and position in labour

Women should be encouraged to achieve the position(s) that they find most comfortable during labour. There are probable advantages to adopting an upright position and for mobilizing during labour. As the nature of their contractions alter, women may find that altering their position will alleviate some of the pain (see Chapter 5). Some women prefer to keep mobile in labour and, when in established labour, may find physical support helpful during contractions. Either continuous or intermittent monitoring can be used under these circumstances.

TABLE 3-1. MINIMUM FREQUENCY OF OBSERVATIONS IN NORMAL LABOUR

Observation	Frequency
Temperature	4-hourly if normal
Blood pressure	2-hourly if normal
Pulse	2-hourly
Fetal heart	Auscultation with fetal stethoscope or Doppler every 15–30 min
	Auscultation with fetal stethoscope or Doppler after every contraction or every 5 min in the second stage
Colour of amniotic fluid	At each vaginal examination once membranes have ruptured
Urine	Encouraged to empty bladder 2-hourly. Urinalysis performed on admission only or more frequently if indicated
Uterine contractions (duration and frequency)	hourly
Abdominal palpation	4-hourly
Vaginal examination	4-hourly

Eating and drinking in normal labour
Withholding food and drink from women in normal labour is unlikely to be beneficial. The woman's appetite should be a guide as to what she wants to eat and drink. If circumstances change and particularly if a Caesarean section is likely, then only small amounts of fluid should be offered. Excessive drinking has occasionally been associated with neonatal hyponatraemia.

Pain relief
Individual women will have differing attitudes towards the use of pain relieving methods/drugs in labour. Some women will be quite definite about what they wish to happen, others will be less so. Antenatal education should help women to make decisions, but not all women attend

classes. The person(s) caring for the woman should encourage and help her with the chosen method(s) and when appropriate give her advice/information on alternatives should the need be apparent. Chapter 5 deals with methods of pain relief, including epidural analgesia.

Complimentary therapies

If a woman takes any homeopathic or other 'natural' remedies during the course of her labour a record of the time, dosage and name of the substance should be made in her records. It must be made clear that the woman takes these remedies at her own responsibility.

THE SECOND STAGE OF LABOUR

The second stage of labour is usually diagnosed when the woman has an overwhelming urge to push and is fully dilated or the presenting part is visible. If the second stage is diagnosed on vaginal examination, pushing should be commenced only when the woman has the urge and should not be encouraged before this time. A vaginal examination should always be performed if, soon after the urge to push, there are no clear signs of the second stage.

At the onset of the second stage of labour, the resuscitaire and equipment for neonatal resuscitation in the room should be checked. If adequate equipment is not available, the midwife in charge of labour ward should be informed.

The woman should be encouraged to adopt the most comfortable position she can achieve and be well supported by pillows if appropriate. Upright positions are more beneficial than supine positions.

The midwife caring for the woman should be the person advising the woman during the second stage.

The woman's blood pressure should be measured at the onset of the second stage, and if normal, every 30 min during the active phase. If blood pressure is 140/100 or above, the SHO should be informed and the blood pressure monitored every 15 min and the urine checked at the next opportunity.

If continuous CTG monitoring is not in progress, the fetal heart should be listened to after every contraction. All values should be recorded. If the auscultated fetal heart rate (FHR) gives cause for concern, then a continuous record of the FHR should be obtained using an electronic fetal monitor (EFM)

The obstetric SHO or specialist registrar should be informed if the delivery is not thought to be imminent after the woman has been push-

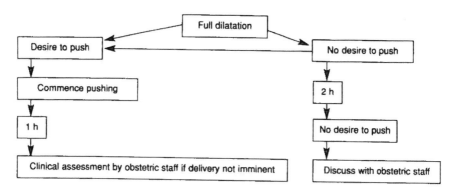

FIGURE 3-1. Management of second stage of labour in women without an epidural (assuming normal CTG)

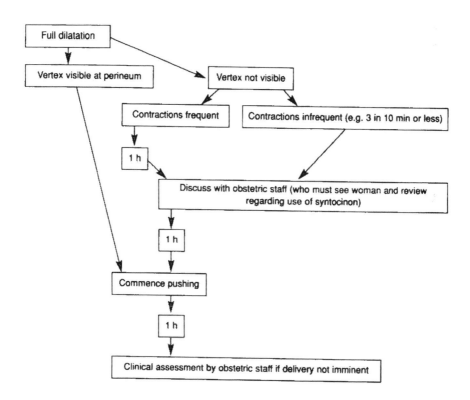

FIGURE 3-2. Management of second stage of labour in women with an epidural (assuming normal CTG)

29

ing for more than 1 h. If the SHO makes the initial assessment at this time, the SHO must discuss the case with the specialist registrar on call.

If a woman has an epidural, pushing need not commence until the presenting part is visible or after full dilatation for 2 h. Full dilatation must be confirmed by vaginal examination. For management of second stage of labour see flowcharts.

Episiotomy

This subject should be discussed with the woman in the antenatal period and/or in early labour so that she is aware of the circumstances in which an episiotomy may be necessary. The decision as to whether an episiotomy is needed will be made by the person conducting the delivery. The most common indications for performing an episiotomy are an instrumental delivery or if fetal compromise is suspected.

Female genital mutilation

If female genital mutilation is newly diagnosed in labour, please see Chapter 28.

Meconium-stained liquor

The amount of liquor and thickness of meconium should be clearly recorded in the notes at each vaginal examination. At delivery, every attempt should be made to aspirate meconium from the oropharynx as soon as possible (e.g. at the perineum for vaginal delivery and on the table at Caesarean section). However, if the baby needs urgent paediatric attention, then priority should be given to passing the baby to the attendant paediatricians.

THIRD STAGE OF LABOUR

Whether the third stage is managed physiologically or actively, signs of separation must be awaited before delivering the placenta[3,4]. Signs of separation are a trickle of blood at the introitus, the uterus becoming smaller, narrower and rounder, and cord lengthening[5].

Evidence from a well-conducted randomized trial indicates that active management reduces the risk of postpartum haemorrhage (PPH)[4]. However, decisions about individual care should take into account the weight placed by pregnant women and their caregivers on PPH and blood transfusion compared with an intervention-free third stage after a straightforward labour. For women having a waterbirth, it is recommended that they leave the pool for the delivery of the placenta, as it is often difficult to estimate blood loss.

Women at low risk of PPH who opt for physiological management of the third stage, based on informed choice, should be told that the management will change if they start to haemorrhage, as the woman's safety takes precedence.

It is recommended that women with a history of the following should not have a physiological third stage:

- placenta praevia

- previous PPH due to uterine atony

- antepartum haemorrhage

- anaemia (haemoglobin < 9 g/dl or mean corpuscular volume < 75 fl)

- instrumental delivery

- prolonged first or second stage

- multiple pregnancy

- intrauterine death

- epidural anaesthesia

- parity > 5

- large uterine fibroids

- oxytocin infusion

- anticoagulant therapy

- chorioamnionitis

- polyhydramnios

TABLE 3-2. MANAGEMENT OF THE PHYSIOLOGICAL THIRD STAGE OF LABOUR

- No prophylactic oxytocic drug to be given
- Encourage the mother to breastfeed if she wishes
- If possible, leave the cord attached to the baby until the placenta is delivered
- No controlled cord traction
- Instruct the mother to concentrate on feeling the next contraction or an urge to push. Women who do not have syntocinon should be warned that the contractions in the third stage of labour may be quite mild and they should be asked to bear down, even during the mildest of pains, to aid the birth of the placenta

Continued

TABLE 3-2. (continued)

- When the mother feels a contraction or there are signs of separation (including the cord no longer pulsating), encourage her to adopt a position she finds comfortable that will aid the effect of gravity and encourage expulsion of the placenta by maternal effort. Once the placenta is in the vagina, the cord may be used to guide the placenta out gently
- If the placenta does not deliver spontaneously, wait and reattempt expulsion by maternal effort with gravity
- If the woman intends to breastfeed, this is an ideal time for the baby to feed as feeding will aid expulsion of the placenta

---

TABLE 3-3. SPECIAL CIRCUMSTANCES IN THE MANAGEMENT OF THE PHYSIOLOGICAL THIRD STAGE OF LABOUR

- Need to clamp and cut the cord before placental delivery – e.g. meconium-stained liquor or if the cord is around baby's neck. Blood should be released from placental end into a kidney dish, and the cord left unclamped
- Rhesus-negative mothers – if cord clamping has been necessary, take cord bloods as soon as possible before releasing the placental end
- If there is no blood in the cord, fetal blood can be obtained from vessels on the placental surface near cord insertion
- Placenta undelivered after 1 h – ensure the woman has emptied her bladder; attempt delivery by maternal effort; manage actively (bolus of oxytocic drug and controlled cord traction). If placenta still undelivered after further 15 min, seek advice of senior midwife or obstetrician
- In all circumstances (e.g. serious blood loss), the safety of the mother takes precedence

---

Active management of the third stage

Intramuscular syntometrine 1 ml (1 ampoule) or syntocinon 10 IU should be given as soon as possible after delivery of the anterior shoulder. Clamp and cut the cord as soon as possible after delivery of the baby. After cord blood has been taken, the clamp from the maternal end may be released if wished. The mother may be encouraged to breastfeed the baby if she wishes.

After signs of placental separation, the mother should be encouraged to adopt a semirecumbent position and deliver the placenta by controlled cord traction. The rate of PPH may be increased when CCT is used without awaiting signs of separation[6].

SPECIAL CIRCUMSTANCES

If the placenta is undelivered after 30 min, ensure that the mother's bladder is empty. Delivery should be attempted by gentle controlled cord traction or maternal effort with or without gravity. If the placenta is still undelivered, advice of senior midwife or obstetrician should be sought. Controlled cord traction should never be applied at the same time as maternal effort or gravity assistance.

In all circumstances (e.g. serious blood loss), the safety of the mother and baby takes precedence.

The immediate post-partum period

Immediately following delivery the baby should be located in a place according to the mother's wishes. Some women may wish to hold the baby immediately after birth, others may want a delay. The baby should then be dried and covered with a warm dry towel. The necessary observations of the mother and baby should be made in a non-intrusive way, allowing the woman and her partner to focus on the first moments with their child.

Suturing the perineum

If the perineum requires suturing this should be done as soon as possible by a person with the relevant training, preferably within 1 h of delivery. The person who delivers the baby or conducts the delivery should preferably perform the suturing to allow continuity of care[7]. The procedure should be explained to the mother and the woman's wishes must also be taken into consideration.

Midwives may undertake suturing of the perineum providing that they have undertaken the appropriate training. This includes:

- a formal lecture on the practical techniques used for the repair, and

- undertaking a minimum of six repairs under the guidance of an experienced midwife or doctor

Following this training, it is for the midwife in conjunction with a senior midwife or supervisor of midwives to confirm that she is competent to undertake the procedure. If the midwife herself is in doubt that she is competent to perform suturing, she should seek further advice from her senior midwife or supervisor.

Polyglactin remains the material of choice for repair of all the tissue layers. Its use is associated with about 40% reduction in short-term pain and the need for analgesia[8]. The continuous subcuticular technique appears preferable to interrupted transcutaneous suturing, causing less perineal pain in the early puerperium[9].

Suturing the vaginal mucosa and muscle layers, but leaving the skin unsutured, may be associated with reduced pain postpartum and no increased risk of breakdown of the repair and resuturing[10]. Suturing two layers rather than three is not the same as leaving the second-degree tear unsutured.

There is no satisfactory randomized controlled trial evidence comparing suturing and non-suturing of second-degree tears. Second-degree tears should be sutured. If the woman makes an informed choice not to have a second-degree tear sutured, this should be clearly documented in the clinical records.

When all the equipment is ready, the mother should be placed in the lithotomy position ensuring both legs are raised together. Ensure that the legs are not abducted excessively. In women with pubic symphysitis, suturing should be performed using a narrow table, e.g. that in theatres. Where the lithotomy position is not possible, for example at a home birth, the woman can lie on a bed with her buttocks at the edge of the bed and her legs wide apart with her feet on chairs.

TABLE 3-4. EQUIPMENT FOR PERINEAL SUTURE PACK

Lignocaine 1%
20-ml syringe
Green or blue needle
Vicryl Rapide (polyglactin) or similar dissolvable suture(s)
Warm sterile water
Obstetric cream
Gloves
Lithotomy poles
A good light/spotlight
Entonox

The repair is carried out using aseptic conditions under a good light. Use gauze to clear away blood and fluid from the field of vision. During the procedure use swabs to clear away any ooze rather than try and insert a large ready-made taped tampon into the vagina. If a tampon is inserted, a clip should be attached to the tail of the tampon. A maternity pad or gauze must never be used in place of a tampon – they may be forgotten and left inside the vagina, resulting in infection. If the taped tampon is used, moisten the tampon with a little obstetric cream before insertion.

TABLE 3-5. PRINCIPLES OF GOOD SUTURING

- Avoid using too many sutures, but use enough to ensure haemostasis and alignment of tissues
- Allow for physiological oedema – the sutures should not be too tight as suturing too tightly causes more pain later
- Wipe wound free of clots, and beware of losing cut ends of suture material in the wound

Difficult repairs e.g. where there has been female genital mutilation (FGM), cervical tears, extensive vaginal tearing, tears involving the urethra or a third-degree tear are referred to the obstetric specialist registrar. If in doubt, consult a more senior midwife or obstetrician.

Pain relief

Women who have an effective epidural analgesia may not require lignocaine. Midwives should consult their current standing orders before using lignocaine. At the time of print, a midwife can use a maximum of 20 ml of 1% lignocaine to infiltrate the perineum. When doing so, pay most attention to the sensitive introitus. The mother may use entonox during infiltration and in addition to lignocaine during the suturing if she wishes. Three minutes should be allowed before commencing suturing to enable the lignocaine to work. Test for numbness prior to suturing to confirm effectiveness of the lignocaine.

Technique

Any bleeding point should be noted after delivery and tied off separately by lifting with forceps and tying a loop of suture material around it. If haemostasis cannot be achieved, an obstetrician should be called.

The apex of the episiotomy/tear should be clearly identified. The first suture should be placed above the apex of the episiotomy/tear and tied three times. The posterior vaginal wall is then closed with a continuous suture. Sutures should be placed approximately 0.5 cm from the edge of the wound, 1 cm apart and 0.5 cm deep (remembering the proximity of rectum). The sutures are continuously inserted until the introitus is reached using the hymen ring remnants as a landmark. A loop of the final suture is left so a firm knot can be tied three times to complete the closure of the posterior vaginal wall and reconstruct the introitus. The ends of the suture are trimmed to about 0.5 cm.

The perineal body is now closed with interrupted sutures, going from front to back for easier apposition of tissues. The depth of the episiotomy/tear must be defined.

Continuous subcuticular sutures are used along the muscle layer at approximately half the depth. In the event of a very deep episiotomy/ tear, the muscle layer may need two lines of sutures at different depths.

A line of sub-cuticular continuous sutures (or interrupted sutures in some cases, for example in a very ragged tear) now closes the skin going from back to front or top to bottom. The knots are buried to be more comfortable for the woman.

Completion

The tampon (if used) is removed and the vagina is checked, i.e. if it easily admits two fingers, the line of the sutures is competent and no swabs or gauze are *in situ*.

The rectum is examined by inserting the little finger lubricated with obstetric cream to check that no sutures have penetrated through from the repair. If so, remove the suture and inform the obstetric specialist registrar.

The mother's perineum is swabbed clean, and a maternity pad is applied to the vulva. Needles and swabs should be counted and disposed of correctly. Extra blood loss at this stage is added to the total in the mother's notes.

Prior to vacating the delivery room, the resuscitaire and equipment for neonatal resuscitation should be checked and restocked

Record keeping

The repair is recorded in the mother's notes, illustrated with a diagram for clarity if necessary. The operator should always sign using full signature, followed by name in capitals, date and time.

For example:

Suturing of a second degree tear. Infiltration of perineum and perineal body with 20 ml of 1% lignocaine. Continuous vicryl to posterior vaginal wall, interrupted to muscle and sub-cuticular to skin.

Haemostasis achieved.

Tampon removed.

P.V. and P.R. - N.A.D.

S/M Josephine Bloggs
JOSEPHINE BLOGGS
16 July 1999

SUTURE OF A THIRD-DEGREE TEAR

Suturing a third-degree tear should always be performed or supervised by the senior specialist registrar on call, who should explain the complication and its significance to the patient. The surgery should be performed in the labour ward theatre. The edges of the anal sphincter should be visualized in total and brought together and sutured with two to four interrupted sutures under direct vision using PDS or similar suture material. The rectal mucosa should be sutured with interrupted sutures and the knots tied externally (i.e. protruding into the anal canal). Laxatives should be prescribed and arrangements made for postnatal 6 week follow-up by obstetric staff.

BABY EXAMINATION

When the baby is initially examined by the midwife in the delivery room, it is essential that the purpose, nature and outcome of the examination are explained to the parents. It is also important that the baby's identity bracelets are attached as soon as possible following delivery. Two labels should be applied, one around each ankle. Written on them should be the mother's full name, her hospital number, the sex of the baby, the baby's number and the date and time of the birth. The labels must always be checked with the mother (or partner if she is not able).

The mother will stay on the labour ward until her observations are stable prior to her transfer to the postnatal ward.

Before transfer, mother and baby should be made clean and comfortable. The mother and partner should be offered something to eat and drink. If the mother wishes to breastfeed, ensure that the baby has the opportunity to be put to the breast within the first hour after delivery or, if artificial feeding is the chosen method and the baby appears hungry, a feed may be offered whilst still on the labour ward.

The mother is normally transferred to the postnatal ward in a wheelchair with her baby in her arms. She should be transported on a bed if she has had an epidural. The midwife or student midwife who attended the mother at delivery should normally accompany her and give the handover report to the midwife on the ward. The notes and computer printout should accompany the mother. In exceptional circumstances, if the printout is not complete, a handwritten information sheet should be completed and accompany the mother. The birth notification or handwritten or computer-generated sheet should be signed by the midwife responsible and left on labour ward.

REFERENCES

1. Mires G, Williams F, Howie P. Randomised controlled trial of cardiotocography versus Doppler ausculation of fetal heart at admission in labour in low-risk obstetric population. *Br Med J* 2001;322:1457-60
2. *The Use of Electronic Fetal Monitoring: the Use and Interpretation of Cardiotocography in Intrapartum Fetal Surveillance* (Guideline no. 8J. London: RCOG Press, 2001
3. Levy V. The midwife's management of the third stage of labour. In: Alexander J, Levy V, Roch S, eds. *Midwifery Practice: Intrapartum Care – A Research-Based Approach*. Basingstoke, UK: Macmillan, 1990
4. Rogers J, Wood J, McCamdlish R, *et al.* Active versus expectant management of third stage of labour: the Hinchingbrooke randomised controlled trial. *Lancet* 1998;351:693-9
5. Morrin N. Midwifery care in the third stage of labour. In: Sweet B, Tiran D, eds. *Mayes' Midwifery, a Textbook for Midwives*, 12th edn. London: Bailliere Tindall, 1997
6. Levy V, Moore J. The midwife's management of the third stage of labour. *Nursing Times* 1985;81:47-50
7. Cunningham A. Perineal damage in childbirth. *Nursing Mirror* 1984;158 (suppl):i-ix
8. Grant A. The choice of suture materials and techniques for repair of perineal trauma: an overview of the evidence from controlled trials. *Br J Obstet Gynaecol* 1996;96:1281-9
9. Chalmers I, Enkin M, Keirse MJNC. *Effective Care in Pregnancy & Childbirth*, Vol 2. Oxford, UK: Oxford University Press, 1989.
10. Gordon B, Mackrodt C, Fern E, Truesdale A, Ayers S, Grant A. The Ipswich Childbirth Study: 1. A randomised evaluation of two stage postpartum perineal repair leaving the skin unsutured. *Br J Obstet Gynaecol* 1998;105:435-40

BIBLIOGRAPHY

Clements RV. *Safe Practice in Obstetrics and Gynaecology*. Edinburgh, UK: Churchill Livingstone, 1994:492

Edmonds DK, ed. *Dewhurst's Textbook of Obstetrics and Gynaecology for Postgraduates*, 6th edn. Oxford, UK: Blackwell Science, 1999:622

James DK, *et al.* High Risk Pregnancy. London: WB Saunders, 1994:1318

4

The unbooked woman presenting to the labour ward

The unbooked woman presenting to the labour ward should be admitted under the consultant on call at that time. The midwife should admit the woman and determine whether she has attended any hospital previously. The midwife should complete an admission form and then telephone the administrative department to obtain a hospital number.

It is important to establish when possible why the labouring woman is unbooked. In general, such women are high risk, and the likely reason in each case may have an important influence on care. Where relevant, the immigration status should be checked and the care arrangements of the woman's other children should be established (if she has them). Staff should always check any social services documentation available.

All booking blood tests must be done, after informed consent (full blood count [FBC], group and antibody, random blood sugar [if 28 weeks' gestation or more], rubella, hepatitis B and C, *Treponema pallidum* haemagglutination assay/Venereal Disease Research Laboratory test and HIV testing). The FBC, blood group and sickle cell results should be obtained urgently. If the woman delivers prior to the blood results being available, cord blood should be taken for a Coombs' test and FBC.

The senior house officer (SHO) on call should see the woman and, after taking a full social, medical/surgical and obstetric history, inform the specialist registrar who should review the woman and formulate the care plan. If the woman is not in labour and she intends to deliver at the hospital, an urgent booking appointment should be arranged in the antenatal clinic. If the woman has a primary care physician, inform him/her and obtain any further relevant information.

An ultrasound (US) scan should be performed to check fetal well-being, presentation and placental position. A vaginal examination should not be performed until the placenta has been shown to be not low on US.

WOMEN BOOKED AT ANOTHER HOSPITAL

If the labouring woman has notes, she should be admitted as per the labour ward admission protocol (being seen by SHO/specialist registrar if required). If the woman is in labour and recent blood results are not available, blood must be taken and sent as urgent specimens for FBC and blood group. Other bloods should be taken as required. If the woman delivers before the blood result is available, cord blood should be taken for Coombs' testing and FBC.

The hospital in which the woman is booked should be contacted and informed that she has been admitted and that she has or will be delivering at an alternate hospital. There may be other relevant information about the woman that is not in her handheld notes.

The various social services documentation available in the maternity unit should be checked for details of the woman.

If the patient does not have notes, she should be admitted as per labour ward protocol following the protocol for unbooked women. The hospital at which she is booked must be telephoned in order to obtain any relevant information and, if the woman is in labour, request that a record of her notes and blood results be faxed.

If in labour, blood tests need to be undertaken for FBC and blood group. Results must be sent back to the labour ward urgently. Other booking bloods may be taken as required. If the woman delivers before the results for blood group are available, cord blood should be taken for Coombs' testing and FBC.

Risk management

It is advisable that a multidisciplinary assessment needs to be made when either unbooked women or women who are booked for delivery in another hospital request early discharge.

BIBLIOGRAPHY

Clements RV. *Safe Practice in Obstetrics and Gynaecology*. Edinburgh: Churchill Livingstone, 1994:492

5

Pain relief in labour

INTRODUCTION

Many factors will influence the way in which a woman is able to or wishes to cope with pain in labour. It is possible in most units to provide a woman with a wide range of pain-relieving methods, and it is likely that she may wish to use more than one method during the course of her labour.

It is essential that every woman is given as much information as possible about the options that are available and supported in her choice.

Before considering the pharmacological methods that are available, it is worth considering other factors that may influence either the amount of pain that a woman feels or the amount that she feels able to cope with without medication.

POSTURE AND POSITIONS IN LABOUR

During the course of labour, the woman may find that by adopting different positions she is able to relieve some of the pressure and pain. If she has been to antenatal preparation classes, she may be very familiar with these positions and be able to adopt them with minimal help. Other women may not have attended such classes or may not remember all they were shown. It is important that staff caring for the women are familiar with alternative positions and feel confident enough to encourage the women to adopt them.

WATER LABOUR AND WATER BIRTH

There is no doubt water can have a beneficial effect on pain. Many women find being in water during the first stage of labour helpful. Unless the labour is high risk, this does not conflict with appropriate fetal surveillance. A few women opt to give birth in water and this is something that is often encouraged in some units, with appropriate guidance.

BIRTH CUSHIONS

Birth cushions are available from a number of sources and even on some labour wards. Some women find them very useful if they wish to adopt a squatting position in labour. Following delivery, the cushions should be washed with the appropriate cleansing solution, dried and stored.

BIRTHING CHAIRS

Modern delivery beds sometimes have the ability to be modified into birthing chairs, which can be helpful to some labouring women.

TRANSCUTANEOUS ELECTRICAL NERVE STIMULATION

Transcutaneous electrical nerve stimulation (TENS) is a method of pain relief that is self-administered. It is freely available for women to buy. Many hospitals organize rental schemes. The woman may bring the apparatus with her when she is in labour. The woman will normally have already been instructed in its use. In this situation, the use of the device is the mother's responsibility, but the midwife should give her any necessary assistance. Previous instruction in the use of TENS is usual and desirable.

Efficacy

In randomized controlled trials, less than 20% of women who used TENS reported good pain relief[1-3]. Pain relief is rarely complete and some women experience no benefit at all[1,4]. Maternal satisfaction is highest when it is used in early labour, possibly because of a placebo effect[5,6].

Side-effects

TENS is generally very safe and free of side-effects, but it may interfere with the cardiotocography (CTG) trace. If so, the medical team should use ultrasound or an external transducer system. TENS is contraindicated if the mother has a pacemaker.

INHALATION ANALGESIA

Entonox is available in the delivery room. It comprises 50% nitrous oxide and 50% oxygen. It is self-administered from a cylinder or piped wall supply with demand valve and mouth piece or face mask.

Inhalation of entonox takes 45–60 s to reach maximum analgesic effect – parturients should be taught to begin inhaling when they first feels a contraction rather than waiting until the contraction becomes painful. Similarly, they should stop inhaling when the peak of the contraction has passed[5].

Efficacy

About three-quarters of women who use entonox in labour find it helpful, although it rarely relieves all of the pain[1]. It generally compares favourably with pethidine and TENS in surveys[1,6].

Side effects and complications

Entonox is generally safe for mother and baby, but there are some mild side effects: central nervous system (CNS) (light-headedness, drowsiness, confusion and disorientation), gastrointestinal (GI) tract (nausea and vomiting) and respiratory system (tends to make women hyperventilate, leading to dizziness, tingling and tetany). There is no evidence of any effect of entonox on labour itself, neither does there seem to be any clinically significant effects on the baby (either fetal or neonatal).

PARENTERAL OPIATES

Intramuscular pethidine

The dose of pethidine given to the labouring woman will vary between 75–150 mg depending on body weight and is decided by the midwife caring for the woman. This may be repeated after a 3 h period if necessary. If a further administration is thought necessary, it must be prescribed by a doctor. If the CTG is normal before the administration of pethidine, then this administration in itself is not an indication for continuous electronic fetal heart rate monitoring. Pethidine alone is never an indication for starting a CTG.

Efficacy
Despite many anecdotal reports and a number of retrospective trials suggesting that pethidine provides satisfactory analgesia, the overwhelming majority of prospective trials continue to report that pethidine is, at best, a poor analgesic in labour[7,8].

Sedation of the mother should not be confused with analgesia[8,9].

Non-analgesic maternal side effects
There are various non-analgesic side effects: CNS (sedation, confusion and respiratory depression) and the GI tract (nausea, vomiting and delayed gastric emptying). Paturients receiving pethidine should also receive ranitidine and metoclopramide to counteract its GI tract side effects[7]. There is no proven side effect of pethidine on progress of labour.

Side-effects in the neonate
Pethidine can cause neonatal respiratory depression, which is most severe if the dose delivery interval is 2–3 h[10]. Naloxone (400 µg/ml, intramuscular dose 0.25 ml/kg [100 µg/kg]) should be available in the delivery room if the mother has received pethidine. Neurobehavioural effects, such as sleepiness, poor sucking and delayed establishment of breastfeeding, may occur[11].

Contraindications
Monoamine oxidase inhibitors (MAOIs) are an absolute contraindication to the use of pethidine. Severe pregnancy-induced hypertension also prohibits the use of pethidine, while norpethidine, an active metabolite, is proconvulsant.

EPIDURAL ANAESTHESIA

In the opinion of women themselves, epidural analgesia generally provides the only reliable form of effective pain relief in labour[12]. However, unless properly managed it provides scope for complications and dissatisfaction.

Epidural anaesthesia is available to any labouring woman who requests it, providing there are no contraindications to its administration. A woman requesting an epidural should be referred to the obstetric anaesthetist who should assess the patient as soon as possible. However, if the on-call anaesthetist is attending another emergency on the labour ward and is not likely to be available to attend to the woman for more than 1 h, then the anaesthetist/midwife should contact the anaesthetic senior specialist registrar to request assistance.

Contraindications

Contraindications to epidural analgesia can be classified as absolute (local or systemic sepsis, significant coagulopathy, patient refusal) or relative (spinal abnormality, hypovolaemia, severe fetal distress, fixed cardiac output states).

Epidural and central blockade may be considered in patients with possible bleeding problems if:

- They are on heparin, low molecular weight heparin or aspirin thromboprophylaxis
- The International Normalized Ratio does not exceed 1.8
- The platelet count is not below $50\ 000 \times 10^9$/ml

and provided that:

- There has been discussion with a senior anaesthetist
- There is no clinically increased bleeding
- The block is performed by an experienced anaesthetist
- Monitoring for signs of spinal cord compression is performed at least every 4 h until 12 h after the removal of the epidural catheter.

ADMINISTRATION OF THE EPIDURAL

The obstetric anaesthetist should offer an explanation to the mother of the following risks of epidural analgesia:

- Headache (< 1%)
- Hypotension
- Failure
- Early local back tenderness
- Itching/shivering

If asked specifically about nerve damage, the anaesthetist should suggest that the risk is very low (< 1 in 13 000)

An intravenous cannula should be inserted prior to epidural analgesia (minimum 16-G) and an intravenous preload of Hartmann's solution

300–500 ml is appropriate in healthy parturients. Sterile preparation should include the anaesthetist wearing gown and gloves.

Details of epidural insertion should be clearly documented on the 'obstetric analgesia chart' by the anaesthetist and this should be filed in the patient's notes. The anaesthetist in UK hospitals is responsible for the first injection of local anaesthetic down the epidural catheter. Midwives may then give subsequent top-ups.

Epidural analgesia should normally be by a 'low-dose' technique (see below). Instructions should be clearly prescribed on the obstetric analgesia chart. After the initial bolus and any subsequent epidural top-up injections, blood pressures should be recorded by the midwife on the reverse side of the obstetric analgesia chart at 5 min intervals for 20 min. During epidural infusions blood pressures should be measured every 30 min.

The anaesthetist should check the efficacy and the sensory level of the block 30 min after the initial epidural dose. Ideally, during epidural infusions, the sensory level should also be checked every hour. The midwife may do this if she has been instructed to do so. With low-dose epidural analgesia, the criteria specified below must be fulfilled before the patient is allowed to ambulate (see page 50).

A urinary catheter will normally be introduced. An epidural may take away the sensation of a full bladder, which may not only prevent descent of the fetal head but may also result in trauma to the bladder. Hands should be washed to prevent infection.

DURAL PUNCTURE

If an accidental dural puncture occurs:

- Epidural analgesia should normally be established in an adjacent lumbar interspace. It may be appropriate to call a senior colleague to do this

- The midwife and patient should be informed of what has occurred. The patient should be counselled about potential problems and management (it may be appropriate to delay this until after analgesia has been established)

- It is unnecessary to perform an elective instrumental delivery unless a headache is already present in labour, therefore pushing at full dilatation should normally be encouraged

- Epidural fluid administration and prophylactic blood patching should not usually be performed

- The patient should be followed up closely by the anaesthetist who caused the complication

- The consultant anaesthetist should be informed and will advise on management

If a postdural puncture headache occurs, management should initially be conservative, but if symptoms persist a blood patch should be performed This should only be done after consultation with a senior obstetric anaesthetist (consultant or senior specialist registrar).

LOW-DOSE EPIDURAL ANALGESIA

The aims of low-dose epidural analgesia are:

- Analgesia without motor block

- Retention of the second stage urge to bear down and the ability to push

- Retention of the sensation of delivery

- Maintenance of bladder sensation and avoidance of urinary retention

- Safety: cardiovascular stability and reduction of effects on fetal heart rate.

Administration of low-dose epidural analgesia
An example of a suitable solution for low-dose epidural analgesia is bupivacaine 0.1% and fentanyl 2 µg/ml. This can be supplied ready mixed in bags direct from the manufacturer. If these are unavailable, the solution can be prepared by the anaesthetist.

The loading epidural dose should be given by an anaesthetist and will normally consist of 10–15 ml of the low-dose mixture. When using this mixture there is no need for a test dose or for divided doses.

Analgesia should then be maintained using the same low-dose mixture. Regimens vary from unit to unit, but can consist of midwife-administered top-ups, patient-controlled epidural anaesthesia or infusions. In the King's College Hospital unit a sophisticated pump is used to provide a combination of a basal infusion with additional patient-controlled boluses. Standard pump settings are:

Basal rate 6 ml/h
Patient-controlled analgesia dose 8 ml
Lockout period 30 min
Hourly limit 22 ml

The standard regimen should be prescribed by the anaesthetist on the obstetric analgesia chart. Only the anaesthetist may alter the pump settings and these changes should also be prescribed on the obstetric analgesia chart.

Top-ups for breakthrough pain or instrumental delivery may also be presented by the anaesthetist, but it should be ascertained that the parturient has been able to make maximum use of the pump regimen before top-ups are administered. These top-ups will normally consist of 0.25% or 0.5 bupivacaine.

Stop the infusion, give no further top-ups and call the anaesthetist if any of the following occur:

- Pulse drops below 60 beats/min

- Respiratory rate drops below 10/min

- Sensory level > T5

- Concern about sedation

- Patient complains of tingling around the mouth

- BP falls below 90 mmHg (also, turn IVI full on and turn woman lateral)

Criteria for allowing sitting out in chair, standing or walking
The patient must be receiving low-dose epidural analgesia and should not normally have received bupivacaine at concentrations greater than 0.1%. The following should be assessed 20 min after any top-up or hourly during an epidural infusion:

- Maternal blood pressure and fetal heart rate should be stable

- Full motor power in the legs (as assessed by straight leg raising under resistance)

- Patient feels subjectively confident to walk

- A midwife is available to support the woman to standing and be by her side constantly during time out of bed

It should be noted that if continuous fetal heart rate monitoring is indicated, the patient may sit in chair or stand by the CTG monitor.

EPIDURAL TOP-UPS BY TRAINED MIDWIVES

A midwife may undertake the topping-up procedure (but not the primary dose through the catheter) providing that the midwife is thoroughly instructed and competent in the technique.

POINTS TO CONSIDER DURING A TOP-UP

The intravenous infusion should be checked, i.e. that it is running. In the event of hypotension, an immediate and rapid intravenous infusion may be lifesaving.

The systolic blood pressure should be checked. If it is below 90 mmHg an anaesthetist should be consulted. A top-up of bupivacaine is likely to reduce the blood pressure. If the blood pressure is low already it may become critically low.

Any written instructions should be checked. These instructions should have been signed by the anaesthetist (drug, dose, quantity and position of mother). Verbal instructions are unacceptable and can lead to errors.

Aspirate, while observing epidural catheter in the region of the puncture site, and look for blood or cerebrospinal fluid in catheter. If there is none, then inject through the filter (to prevent bacterial contamination).

Injection should occur slowly between contractions. The midwife should be aware of any signs or symptoms of light-headedness, tinnitus, nausea, 'pins and needles', twitching or convulsions in the mother, which may indicate an intravenus injection that should be reported immediately to the anaesthetist. Bupivacaine is not injected during a contraction as venous engorgement in the epidural space can increase the height of the block unpredictably.

A detailed record should be kept of the top-up, including the signature of both people checking the drug.

The blood pressure should be monitored and recorded every 5 min for 20 min or longer in the event of hypotension.

All staff should be able to identify what action to take in the event of hypotension: call the anaesthetist; ensure the woman is on her side to prevent supine hypotension; increase intravenous fluids (Hartmann's); give the woman 6 l/min of oxygen; and have ephedrine and saline for injection ready for the anaesthetist to use.

The effectiveness of the top-up should be monitored and recorded, particularly the duration of action and the symmetry of the block, referring to the anaesthetist if it is not effective.

The presence of a working epidural may lengthen the second stage. This is partially as a result of the absence of Ferguson's reflex that normally releases an oxytocic surge, assisting with uterine activity and causing descent and rotation of the presenting part. In women who have a functioning epidural block, spontaneous uterine activity should be allowed to assist in the descent of the presenting part. Until the urge to bear down is present, or the presenting part is visible, pushing should not be initiated and epidural top-ups should continue to be given, if the woman agrees, in order to allow descent of the presenting part (see Chapter 3). If a previously effective epidural becomes ineffective consider whether the cervix may be fully dilated.

REFERENCES

1. Harrison RF, Shore M, Woods T, Mathews G, Gardiner J, Unwin A. A comparative study of TENS, entonox, pethidine + promazine and lumbar epidural for pain relief in labor. *Acta Obstet Gynecol Scand* 1987;66:9–14
2. Howie R. Client controlled pain relief during childbirth. *Midwiv Chronic* 1985;98:294
3. Hughes SC, Daily PA, Partridge C. Transcutaneous nerve stimulation for labor analgesia. *Anesth Analg* 1988;67:S99
4. Nesheim B-I. The use of transcutaneous nerve stimulation for pain relief during labor. *Acta Obstet Gynecol Scand* 1981;60:13–16
5. Wand BE, Wand DR. Calculated kinetics of distribution of nitrous oxide and methoxyflurane during intermittent administration in obstetrics. *Anesthesiology* 1970;32:306–16
6. Holdcroft A, Morgan M. An assessment of the analgesic effect in labour of pethidine and 50% nitrous oxide in oxygen (Entonox). *J Obstet Gynaecol Br Commonw* 1974;81:603–7
7. Barnes J. Pethidine in labour: results in 500 cases. *Br Med J* 1947;5:437–52
8. Olofsson C, Ekblom A, *et al.* Lack of analgesic effect of systemically administered morphine and pethidine on labour pain. *Br J Obstet Gynaecol* 1996; 103:968–72
9. Russell R, Scrutton M, Porter J. *Pain relief in labour*. London: BMJ Publishing group, 1997
10. Shnider S, Moya F. Effects of meperidine on the newborn infant. *Am J Obstet Gynecol* 1964;89:1009–15
11. Weiner PC, Hogg MI, Rosen M. Neonatal respiration, feeding and neurobehavioural state. *Anaesthesia* 1979;34:996–1004
12. Wraight A. Coping with pain. In: Chamberlain G, Wraight A, Steer P, eds. *Pain and its relief in childbirth: the results of a national survey conducted by the National Childbirth Trust*. Edinburgh: Churchill Livingstone, 1993:79–92

6

Use of the birth pool during labour and delivery

INTRODUCTION

The midwife should be willing and confident to undertake the use of a birth pool during a labour under their care. There should always be two midwives present at the delivery. Each midwife should ideally have seen a video on waterbirth and witnessed one delivery. Midwives who have not delivered using a birth pool should be accompanied by a midwife who is experienced. Once that midwife becomes proficient and feels able to cope with emergencies then she will be able to support her colleagues. All midwives should refer to the senior midwife for advice. The senior midwife should also determine if the mother is appropriate for a water birth.

PREPARATION

The request to labour in water normally comes from the woman and her partner, although the midwife may suggest it as a method of pain relief. Water birth should only be considered if it is suggested by the woman.

The woman and her partner should be aware that if there are signs of fetal distress or if labour becomes abnormal the woman will be asked to leave the pool.

Criteria for mothers using the pool

For a water birth, the pregnancy must be uncomplicated and beyond 37 weeks of gestation. If there are doubts about whether the pool should be used for delivery in a particular case then this must be discussed with the senior midwife and medical staff. Mothers should not have had any sedation in the previous 4 h, since there may be difficulty in helping the mother out of the bath in an emergency. Entonox may be used.

Once labour is well established, preparations should be made for the birth:

- A delivery pack should be in readiness
- The neonatal resuscitaire should be available and ready for use
- Warm towels should be available for both mother and baby
- Syntometrine should be on hand

MIDWIVES' GUIDELINES

Labour

The care of women in the first stage of labour should not differ from any other mother in labour who may wish not to be continuously monitored. The maternal and fetal observations should be conducted with the same frequency.

Temperature, pulse and blood pressure should be monitored as with a standard delivery, and abdominal palpation of uterine contractions should occur as normal. Indications for the performing of this procedure should not differ from standard protocols. However, it may be necessary to ask the mother to leave the pool and rest on the bed to facilitate this.

Observations of vaginal loss may be difficult as any loss is diluted in the water. However, observations of blood or heavily meconium-stained liquor would be obvious. The midwife should explain the significance of abnormalities and encourage the mother to leave the pool.

The use of electrical equipment for monitoring the fetal heart rate during water births is contraindicated. A portable Doppler Sonicaid can be used to auscultate the fetal heart before, during and after a contraction with the woman standing out of the water and dried. A cardiotocograph recording of at least 10–20 min can be made every 4 h as an adjunct to intermittent monitoring.

WATER TEMPERATURE

The water temperature during the first stage of labour is primarily dependent on the comfort of the mother. The water may be emptied out and topped up as required to maintain temperature. The temperature for delivery of the newborn must be maintained at 37°C and recorded every 30 min during the second stage.

DELIVERY

Allow the woman to adopt the most comfortable position for herself and to push at her own pace. This allows the perineum to stretch slowly and prevent tearing. Very little control of the head is required unless delivery appears to be occurring very rapidly. It is important that the baby is delivered totally in water – any contact with air may cause it to inhale too soon. Once the head is delivered, the midwife should feel for the cord; if present, it can normally be slipped over the head. The baby will then be born in the usual way. As the baby is born, he or she is gently guided to the surface and placed in the mother's arms with his or her face and nose clear of the surface. Total immersion is to be avoided after birth. Syntometrine should be withheld unless bleeding occurs.

Once the cord has stopped pulsating, it should be clamped and cut, the baby dried and wrapped in a warm dry towel and placed under a heater. The pool is then drained, the mother dried and returned to bed to await delivery of the placenta. The cord clamp should be removed and the cord blood allowed to drain into a bowl.

It can take 20–30 min for the fundus to separate. The midwife should observe the woman, but not interfere with the fundus. Most women will deliver the placenta by maternal effort, or it may need to be gently lifted-out once separation has occurred. Mother and baby are then managed as if it were a normal delivery.

ESTIMATED BLOOD LOSS

Accurate estimation of estimated blood loss (EBL) is difficult. It should be estimated as less than or equal to or as accurately as possible.

PROBLEMS

Cord tightly around the neck
If the cord is very tight around the neck and necessitates clamping prior

to delivery, the mother should be helped into an upright position; clamping must be performed with the perineum and infant's face well clear of the water. Clamping the cord can stimulate breathing movements, which are undesirable when the neonate is underwater.

Shoulder dystocia

Medical staff should be called immediately should shoulder dystocia be suspected. Whilst awaiting their arrival the mother may be lifted into the supported squat position and encouraged to push hard. Alternatively, the mother can be helped into an upright position, with her holding on to the edge of the pool with extra support from her partner. Simultaneously, the bath should be emptied. An episiotomy should then be performed. The squatting position extends the outlet of the pelvis by 30%, so staff should be prepared to deliver the remainder of the baby quickly once the woman is in this position.

Depressed baby

If it appears that the baby is depressed, clamp and cut the cord immediately. The baby should be taken to the resuscitaire, after which management should proceed in the normal way, keeping the baby warm and dry.

Postpartum haemorrhage

In cases of postpartum haemorrhage, clamp and cut the cord and administer 1 ampoule of syntometrine intramuscularly. The mother should then be taken out of the pool and into bed. Management should then proceed according to standard protocols.

7

Care of the baby

INTRODUCTION

After most deliveries, the baby, if the mother wishes, will normally be delivered onto the mother's abdomen and should be dried and well covered with a warm towel. The cord is clamped and cut when appropriate, depending on the management of the third stage of labour or according to the mother's wishes. It is not usually necessary to suction the pharynx and may be harmful if done too vigorously. Most babies do not need suction of the mouth, but if copious blood or mucous is present, this should be performed gently and effectively at birth for 10 s only. Meconium, if present, should also be sucked away. The nostrils should be gently cleared of blood, vernix or mucous by 'blowing the nose' with a swab or tissue. The components of the Apgar score at 1 min and 5 min after birth are recorded as are the times to the first breath and to regular breathing.

If meconium has been noted during labour a paediatrician should be present at delivery. The baby should have suction of the mouth performed at the earliest opportunity, at the perineum for vaginal delivery and on the table for lower segment Caesarean section. However, this should not hinder rapid transfer of the neonate to the neonatal team if the baby needs urgent neonatal care. If the baby is not vigorous at birth, intubation by a paediatrician is appropriate to remove meconium. If the baby is breathing normally, is vigorous and has a normal circulation, the parents can be left to cuddle the baby, apart from intermittent supervision to ensure that all is well.

It is recommended that all babies should receive vitamin K as soon as possible after delivery. The preferred method of administration is via intramuscular injection. Leaflets should be made available to provide mothers and their partners with information. Following vitamin K, the method of administration should be recorded on the patient's notes. The dosages are as follows:

• Babies under 1500 g should receive 0.5 mg intramuscularly

• Babies over 1500 g should receive 1 mg intramuscularly

Oral vitamin K may be given if the parents choose this course after full discussion of the risk involved.

TABLE 7-1. GUIDELINES FOR ADMINISTRATION OF THE ORAL DOSE (ONE ORAL DOSE = 1 mg VITAMIN K)

Breastfed babies 3 doses	Bottle fed babies 1 dose
an oral dose : at birth : 7 days : 4–6 weeks	one oral dose at birth

It is still advised that babies with respiratory depression at birth, instrumental delivery, premature babies of less than 37 weeks' gestation, babies with liver disease or those whose mothers are on anticonvulsant therapy or on warfarin should receive intramuscular vitamin K due to the increased risk of bleeding. This also applies to babies who need to be admitted to the neonatal unit.

Preparations of vitamin K are licensed for intramuscular or oral use. If neonates are breastfed, the first two doses will be given by the midwife and the final dose will be administered by a Health Visitor or primary care physician at the 6-week check-up. It is important to emphasize to the parents that they will need to communicate this to their general practitioner.

ANTICIPATION OF RESPIRATORY DEPRESSION

Respiratory depression is more common in the preterm infant, but may occasionally occur unexpectedly in term births with no obvious predisposing condition. A paediatric senior house officer (SHO) – i.e. a member of the advanced resuscitation team – should be called for such deliveries. When calling the paediatrician, the midwife should do so sooner rather than later and should always state the reason for the call and identify which delivery room is being used. The degree of urgency should also be clearly stated. The following conditions are known to predispose to respiratory depression and are those that more often give rise to acute and sometimes to chronic hypoxia, both of which may occur in the same baby:

- gestation is less than 36 weeks

- presentation is breech or another abnormal presentation

- there is fetal distress and meconium staining, prolapsed cord or antipartum haemorrhage

- delivery is instrumental and is not a low instrumental delivery (i.e. not a 'lift out')

- delivery is by Caesarean section under general anaesthesia

- multiple deliveries (with a specialist registrar if preterm twins and a consultant paediatrician if preterm triplets)

- rhesus antibodies are present

- the obstetrician, anaesthetist or midwife specifically requests a paediatrician because of their specific concern

- there is any other worry about the baby, e.g. suspected abnormality likely to interfere with cardiac or respiratory function

There is no need for paediatricians to be present for elective Caesarean sections that are being performed at 37 weeks' gestation or over for purely maternal reasons unless under general anaesthesia. There is also no need for paediatricians to be present at every low forceps delivery where there is no fetal distress.

The paediatrician must be notified of deliveries of the following groups of infants who, while beyond 36 weeks' gestation, may need review soon after delivery:

- maternal diabetes

- maternal drug dependance and

- prolonged rupture of membranes

UNEXPECTED RESPIRATORY DEPRESSION AT BIRTH

If the baby's breathing is shallow or irregular

After being dried, the baby should be placed in a clean dry warm towel under a radiant heater. The heart rate should be determined by listening to the heart with a stethoscope. If the baby is not breathing, the breathing is irregular, the heart rate is less than 100 or begins to slow, active resuscitation with mask ventilation should be started immediately and the paediatrician called.

If the heart rate is greater than 100 and the baby is well perfused oxygen via a tube can then be placed over the face at 1–2 l/min. The baby should be kept warm and covered and gently stimulated.

Respiratory depression despite ventilation

If respiratory depression persists despite adequate resuscitation and opiates have been given to the mother within 6 h prior to the delivery, naloxone should be administered, unless the mother is an intravenous drug abuser. The dosage is 100 µg/kg intramuscularly, and the preparation is naloxone 400 µg/ml. The baby should be observed carefully to ensure that respiratory depression does not return when the naloxone wears off.

Cessation of breathing after the first few breaths

If a baby who has begun to breathe stops breathing shortly after birth, this is likely to be the result of maternal sedative or analgesic drugs and active resuscitation with mask ventilation should be started immediately and the paediatrician called. Usually low inflation pressures with a mask will suffice, since the lungs are initially inflated by the baby. If the baby fails to respond, naloxone should be considered.

ENDOTRACHEAL INTUBATION

This should only be performed by personnel who are trained and experienced in this method. It should be noted that, if indicated, positive pressure via a mask is likely to achieve effective ventilation if applied properly and can be used before the paediatrician arrives.

MECONIUM ASPIRATION

Babies who have suffered acute or chronic fetal distress may pass meconium. They may also have been stimulated to gasp prior to or during delivery and therefore may inhale meconium. These babies are often stained with meconium, which can also be seen in the nose and mouth. It is imperative that as much meconium should be effectively sucked out of the newborn's oropharynx, nose and trachea as soon as possible after delivery of the head. This meconium should be removed under direct vision via a laryngoscope. Tracheal intubation should also be performed by one of the team experienced in this technique, and meconium aspirated from the trachea. Positive pressure ventilation should be delayed while meconium is being removed. If the heart rate begins to fall and the baby's general condition deteriorates, then ventilation should be commenced immediately following aspiration.

If the liquor is only lightly stained with meconium, and there are no other signs of fetal distress, the baby is unlikely to have inhaled meconium. The nose and mouth should be cleared and the pharynx visualized. If there is no evidence of meconium, intubation will not be necessary.

FIRST MEDICAL EXAMINATION OF THE NEWBORN

The sequence for ensuring a first medical examination of the newborn is as follows:

- The paediatric SHO may undertake it on the next day
- The paediatric SHO may undertake it within 6 h of delivery in women seeking early discharge, if the SHO is not otherwise busy
- If discharged home before seeing a hospital paediatrician, the midwife should discuss the need for the check with the mother and then contact the paediatric outpatient clinic. The mother will need to bring the baby to the clinic for the check-up

If midwives encounter difficulty in contacting the paediatric SHO, they should contact any member of the paediatric team for those babies whose mothers leave hospital within a few hours of birth.

The general practitioner assigned to the newborn may also perform the check, but this possibility should always be discussed with the GP antenatally.

CONCLUSION

In order to become skilled in resuscitation of the newborn and in dealing with emergencies, the steps to be taken should be reviewed repeatedly and the skills involved in resuscitation should be rehearsed and maintained. Neonatal resuscitation courses are often run by hospital neonatal staff, and obstetric staff are recommended to attend these courses when available.

8

Hypoglycaemia in the newborn

NEW UNDERSTANDING ABOUT NEONATAL HYPOGLYCAEMIA IN LOW-RISK INFANTS

Healthy term babies, particularly those who breastfeed on demand, have significantly lower blood glucose concentrations than formula fed babies in the first 2–3 days of life[1]. They also have raised ketone body concentrations, reflecting their ability to mobilize alternative sources of fuel for energy. This is part of the normal physiological adaptation to extrauterine life by the newborn.

Asymptomatic babies of normal weight who are breastfeeding on demand do not need to have their blood glucose measured[2]. A normal range for glucose values in these babies has not been defined and therefore no diagnostic blood glucose level can be set. In addition, the most common method for estimating blood glucose concentration (reagent strips) greatly overestimates 'low' blood sugars. This leads to unnecessary investigation and treatment, as well as distress and loss of confidence for women[3].

ADVERSE SEQUELAE OF HYPOGLYCAEMIA

Prolonged symptomatic hypoglycaemia can cause brain damage, hence the requirement for rapid bedside testing and treatment if there is any possibility that a baby's symptoms are due to hypoglycaemia. There is much more debate regarding the contribution of asymptomatic hypoglycaemia to neurodevelopmental impairment. Data from preterm babies have been interpreted as showing that persistent hypoglycaemia was significantly and independently associated with a worse outcome at 18 months[4]. The study was not specifically designed to examine the effects of hypoglycaemia, and it is possible that the smallest, sickest babies were subjected to more frequent blood sampling and hence had more low values recorded.

BABIES AT INCREASED RISK OF HYPOGLYCAEMIA

Because of their relative inability to mount appropriate metabolic responses to extrauterine life, infants at increased risk of hypoglycaemia require regular feeding in addition to blood glucose monitoring.

SYMPTOMATIC BABIES

If a baby shows any signs of hypoglycaemia (excessive jitteriness, convulsions, apnoea, cyanosis or excessive pallor) blood glucose must be measured regardless of the infant's risk, and the baby's condition urgently reviewed by a paediatrician.

TABLE 8-1. CRITERIA FOR BABIES AT INCREASED RISK OF HYPOGLYCAEMIA

- Baby is less than 37 weeks' gestation
- Birth weight is below the third centile for gestation
- Birth weight is over the 97th centile for gestation
- Apgar score is under 6 at 5 min
- Mother has diabetes (gestational or insulin-dependent)
- Temperature is under 36°C on admission
- Respiration is over 60 per minute
- Colour – cyanosis or excessive pallor
- Muscle tone – excessively floppy

TABLE 8-2. BIRTHWEIGHT CENTILES[5]

Weeks	3rd centile (g)		97th centile (g)	
	Boy	Girl	Boy	Girl
34	1612	1541	2881	2765
35	1786	1712	3159	3032
36	1965	1889	3439	3301
37	2145	2066	3716	3567
38	2323	2243	3985	3824
39	2497	2461	4243	4070
40	2669	2584	4494	4305
41	2842	2748	4744	4531
42	3019	2914	4996	4759

SKIN-TO-SKIN CONTACT AND EARLY FEEDING

All babies can benefit from 'skin-to-skin'. Babies requiring resuscitation at birth can have skin-to-skin as soon as their condition is stable. If the first breastfeed is delayed for any reason, women can be reassured by midwives of the anecdotal evidence that having uninterrupted skin-to-skin contact at a later stage may be of equal benefit.

Babies at increased risk of hypoglycaemia need regular and frequent feeding until demand feeding is established. These babies may be able to breastfeed sufficiently to satisfy their nutritional needs. Staff and parents should be aware of cues from the baby that he/she wants feeding, as this will facilitate the transition to feeding on demand (Table 8-3).

TABLE 8-3. NEONATAL CUES FOR FEEDING

- mouth and tongue movements
- hand-to-mouth movements

Additional feeding cues that the mother should be aware of include:
- rapid eye movements under the eyelids
- hand to hand movements
- body movements
- small sounds (crying is often a sign that these early signals have been missed)

PRETERM AND LOW BIRTH WEIGHT BABIES

Babies will not usually be admitted to postnatal wards unless they are greater than 34 weeks' gestation and over 1850 g. Preterm babies (< 37 weeks) and those who are small for gestational age (below third centile) are at increased risk of harm from hypoglycaemia because of their low glycogen stores, immature gluconeogenic enzymes and relative inability to mount a ketogenic response (mobilize alternative cerebral fuels) to low circulating blood glucose. Blood glucose monitoring is appropriate for these babies even if they are asymptomatic. If a baby shows any signs of hypoglycaemia (excessive jitteriness, convulsions, apnoea, cyanosis or excessive pallor), blood glucose should be measured and the infant's condition urgently reviewed by a paediatrician.

At delivery

All babies should have skin-to-skin contact and an early feed on the labour ward. Routine observations of the baby's temperature, colour, respiration and muscle tone should be recorded.

Provided the baby is otherwise well, however, blood glucose measurement before 3 h is not clinically helpful and may disrupt the first contact between mother and baby and interfere with early feeding.

On the postnatal ward

Infants at increased risk may be able to breastfeed sufficiently to satisfy their nutritional needs. If not, they require supplementation with expressed breast milk (EBM) and/or formula. They should breastfeed when they show signs of hunger, but should not be allowed to wait more than 3 h between feeds[2].

At 3 h after birth record the baby's temperature, colour, respiration, muscle tone and blood glucose level, and ensure the baby has a feed – the amount does not need to be more than 10 ml.

Help the mother to breastfeed (stimulate the baby with skin-to-skin contact and colostrum, and remind the mother about feeding cues). If the baby breastfeeds, assess the quality and duration of the feed and record.

If the baby does not breastfeed effectively help the mother to hand express and give EBM to the infant. If the baby takes EBM record the amount taken. Supplement with formula if the mother cannot express any or sufficient milk.

If the pre-feed glucose level was at or above 2.6 mmol/l, it should be repeated (along with observations) before the next feed in 3 h.

If the pre-feed glucose level was below 2.6 mmol/l, it should be repeated 30–60 min after the feed to ascertain whether hypoglycaemia has been corrected, and if not the paediatrician should be called.

If the pre-feed blood glucose level is below 2.6 mmol/l for two consecutive readings contact the paediatrician for a formal assessment of the baby.

If the blood glucose level has remained 2.6 mmol/l and above for 24 h following delivery, blood glucose testing may be discontinued. Continue to offer the breast/EBM and, if necessary, formula every 3 h and encourage the mother to recognize pre-feeding signs in the baby so that she can move onto demand feeding. The interval between feeds should not exceed 4 h at this stage.

Remember that babies at increased risk can develop problems after the first few days. Continue 3–4-hourly feeding and observations of the baby's vital signs. The schedule of observations can be reviewed on a daily basis and discontinued as appropriate.

Use the precision-G analyzer on the postnatal ward. If this is not available, take 0.1 ml of the baby's blood in a yellow fluoride tube to the neonatal ward and ask the staff to process it. Do not use BM reagent strips to test babies' blood glucose levels. They have poor sensitivity and specificity for newborns.

INFANT OF A DIABETIC MOTHER

Infants of diabetic mothers are at increased risk of harm from hypoglycaemia because they may become hyperinsulinaemic following delivery, causing a rebound hypoglycaemia. The risk is highest in the macrosomic infants of mothers whose diabetes has been poorly controlled.

Blood glucose monitoring is appropriate for these babies even if they are asymptomatic.

If a baby shows any signs of hypoglycaemia (excessive jitteriness, convulsions, apnoea, cyanosis or excessive pallor) blood glucose should be measured and the infant's condition urgently reviewed by a paediatrician.

At delivery

All babies should have skin-to-skin contact and an early feed on the labour ward.

Routine observations of the baby's temperature, colour, respiration and muscle tone should be recorded.

Provided the baby is otherwise well, however, blood glucose measurement before 3 h is not clinically helpful and may disrupt the first contact between mother and baby and interfere with early feeding.

On the postnatal ward

At 3 h after birth, record the baby's temperature, colour, respiration, muscle tone and blood glucose level. If the pre-feed glucose level at 3 h after delivery is normal (at least 2.6 mmol/l) it is unlikely that supplements will be required, although pre-feed blood glucose measurement should continue 3-hourly for the first 24 h. If the level is below 2.6 mmol/l at 3 h, the baby will need supplements of EBM or, if necessary, formula for 24–48 h. Feeding management is similar to other at-risk groups (see above).

TABLE 8-4. HYPOGLYCAEMIA GUIDELINES FOR BABIES AT LOW RISK

Low-risk criteria
Baby is 37 weeks' gestation and above
Birth weight > 3rd centile for gestation
Birth weight < 97th centile for gestation
Apgar > 6 at 5 min
No maternal diabetes (gestational or insulin dependent)

Plus the baby has normal:
- Temperature (36–37.5°C)
- Colour
- Muscle tone
- Respiration (< 60 per min)

Figure 8-1. outlines care for the low-risk baby in the early postnatal period in hospital.

Review the feeding history of all low-risk babies at 8 h after delivery. Check the notes for the quality of the first feed. Record your actions at all stages of the flow chart

IF the baby has not fed in the last 4 h

Gently rouse and stimulate the baby with skin-to-skin contact, colostrum on mother's nipple/areola/baby's lips. Offer the breast. If the baby is not interested in feeding show the mother how to hand express and remind her about her baby's feeding cues. If expressed milk is obtained, it can be given to the baby in a cup by staff who have received appropriate training or by bottle with maternal consent. Note the amount taken

If the baby takes some colostrum continue to help mother hand express and to remind her about baby's feeding cues. Observe the next feed. Reassess the situation after 8 h

If the baby shows no interest in feeding and has no colostrum, check its colour, muscle tone, respiration and temperature. If these are within normal limits, leave the baby to rest. Reassess the situation after 4 h. If the baby cannot be roused s/he may be unwell and needs paediatric review

If in this time the baby has not fed, check colour, muscle tone, respiration and temperature. If these are normal, rouse and stimulate the baby as above and offer the breast. If the baby is not interested in feeding help the mother to hand express colostrum. This can be given to the baby in a cup by staff who have received appropriate training or by bottle with maternal consent. Note the amount taken

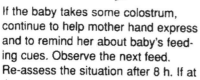 

If the baby takes some colostrum, continue to help mother hand express and to remind her about baby's feeding cues. Observe the next feed. Re-assess the situation after 8 h. If at that time the baby has not fed again repeat Step 3

If a baby has shown no interest in feeding or had any colostrum by 12 h s/he may be unwell, and should be reviewed by a paediatrician.

If at any time the baby's colour, muscle tone, respiration or temperature become abnormal or s/he is excessively jittery or difficult to rouse, ALERT THE PAEDIATRICIAN

FIGURE 8-1 Care for the low-risk baby in the early postnatal period

REFERERENCES

1. Hawdon JM, Ward Platt MP, Aynsley-Green A. Patterns of metabolic adaptation for preterm and term infants in the first neonatal week. *Arch Dis Child* 1992;67:356–65
2. Williams AF. *Hypoglycaemia of the Newborn.* Geneva: World Health Organisation, 1997
3. Dodds R, Newburn M. Low blood glucose an NCT investigation. *Mod Midwife* 1996:14–17
4. Lucas A, Morley R, Cole TJ, Adverse neurodevelopmental outcome of moderate neonatal hypoglycaemia. *Br Med J* 1988;257:1304–6
5. Cole TJ. Birthweight and head circumference centiles. In: Rennie JM, Roberton NRC, eds. *Textbook of Neonatology*, 3rd edn. Edinburgh: Churchill Livingstone, 1999:1404–7

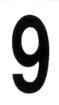

Breastfeeding on labour ward and skin-to-skin contact

INTRODUCTION

Early, exclusive, unrestricted and effective breastfeeding meets a baby's nutrient and fluid requirements. This assumes that the establishment and maintenance of breastfeeding is properly managed at all stages.

BACKGROUND AND EVIDENCE

Benefits of early contact combined with early breastfeeding have been shown for:

- the duration of breastfeeding[1]
- the relationship between mother and baby[2] and
- the baby's core temperature[3]

The benefits of skin-to-skin contact alone are that it:

- helps babies maintain their body temperature better compared to wrapped in a blanket in a cot[4]

- helps babies and their mothers initiate breastfeeding more success-fully than those who do not (uninterrupted skin-to-skin contact)[5]

The effects of labour ward routines include;

- disruption of skin-to-skin contact immediately after birth causing dis-organized feeding behaviour[5,6]

- delays in suckling and shorter duration of breastfeeding associated with pethidine use during labour[5,7,8]

TABLE 9-1. CURRENT RECOMMENDATIONS FOR SKIN-TO-SKIN CONTACT[9]

- Early skin-to-skin contact between mother and baby should be offered as standard care by staff, both antenatally and in labour. Women may choose not to have skin-to-skin contact, and their wishes should be respected
- The period of skin-to-skin should be prolonged (minimum 30 min) and should not be limited or interrupted by procedures that can wait (e.g. weighing, washing and wrapping the infant) unless the mother specifically requests these be done
- Skilled assistance should be available when the baby shows s/he is ready to feed
- Women should be informed antenatally of the possible adverse effect that pethidine in labour may have on the baby's ability to feed at birth and in the subsequent hours and days after birth
- There is little evidence for a 'critical period' during which time women must initiate breastfeeding. Therefore, if the initiation of breastfeeding is unavoidably delayed, women should be reassured that having uninter-rupted skin-to-skin contact at a later stage may be of equal benefit

---

The UNICEF UK Baby Friendly Initiative Step 4 encourages the initia-tion of breastfeeding soon after birth. Uninterrupted skin-to-skin contact allows the infant to express a range of behaviour signs including that s/he is ready to feed (e.g. sucking and rooting, hand-to-mouth and body movements[6]). Strenuous efforts to feed a baby before he/she is ready may disrupt this process, contribute to faulty sucking technique and be counter-productive[10,11]. This is one of the reasons that the Baby Friendly Initiative now prioritize skin-to-skin contact, with feeding as soon as the infant shows he/she is ready.

SKIN-TO-SKIN CONTACT AND EARLY FEEDING

All babies, regardless of intended method of feeding, should have the opportunity to have skin-to-skin contact and to have their first feed soon after delivery.

The majority of babies will show interest in feeding in the first few hours following birth, especially if the mother and baby have had the opportunity of skin-to-skin contact. Staff and parents should be aware of cues from the baby that he/she wants feeding: sucking and rooting movements and hand to mouth movements

Additional feeding cues that the mother should be aware of include: rapid eye movements under the eyelids, hand-to-hand movements, body movements and small sounds (crying is often a sign that these early signals have been missed).

DISCUSSION ABOUT SKIN-TO-SKIN CONTACT

If it has not happened antenatally, discussion of skin-to-skin contact procedure should occur on admission to labour ward, highlighting:

- The benefits of skin-to-skin contact for all infants

- What will happen after delivery. Explain that weighing the baby will ideally be delayed, unless the mother requests otherwise. Describe the circumstances where skin-to-skin contact may be delayed – e.g. if the baby requires resuscitation

- The woman's preferences

All mothers need effective and knowledgeable support with the initiation of breastfeeding, but the following may need extra help to establish breastfeeding:

- Babies whose mothers had pethidine in labour
- Babies whose mothers are on certain medications (e.g. anticonvulsants)
- Babies whose mothers have had a Caesarean section
- Babies whose mothers have had a general anaesthetic
- Mothers who have had breastfeeding problems in the past

SKIN-TO-SKIN CONTACT AND EARLY FEEDING AFTER DELIVERY

Skin-to-skin contact keeps babies warm. Infants who have uninterrupted skin-to-skin contact immediately after birth show a range of behaviour including cues that he/she is ready to feed. Skin-to-skin contact and early effective feeding also promote successful breastfeeding (initiation and duration). Whatever their feeding intention, all mothers should have the opportunity for an unhurried period of skin-to-skin contact with their baby after delivery. Women should be informed of the possible adverse effects of pethidine on infant feeding and that the period of skin-to-skin contact should not be interrupted by procedures that can wait (e.g. weighing, washing, neonatal exam). If the mother specifically request it, the period of skin-to-skin contact can start after these procedures.

TABLE 9-2. FOLLOWING NORMAL DELIVERY* OF A BABY THAT DOES NOT REQUIRE RESUSCITATION**

- Gently dry the baby
- Place the baby in skin-to-skin contact with the mother (on her abdomen/between her breasts)
- Put a warmed towel/blanket over the baby and mother
- Complete third stage (if this hasn't already happened) and check maternal fundus and blood loss
- Leave mother and baby to get acquainted asking her to buzz if the baby looks like he/she wants to feed
- Check on the mother and baby after examining the placenta
- Ideally, the mother should be able to remain like this in an unhurried environment for as long as she chooses and for at least 30 min

* Following Caesarean section, women should be given their babies to hold with skin-to-skin contact within 30 min of the baby being able to respond
** Following effective resuscitation the baby may be given to the mother at any stage, unwrapped and placed in skin-to-skin contact

EARLY FEEDING

Assist with the first feed (breast or bottle) as soon as the baby is ready. The majority of babies will show interest in feeding if the mother and baby have had the opportunity of skin-to-skin contact. Staff and parents should be aware of cues from the baby that he/she wants feeding (sucking and rooting movements and hand-to-mouth movements, and in the absence of assistance, finding the nipple and starting to suckle spontaneously). As soon as pre-feeding signs are exhibited, assistance with the first feed should be offered. It should be noted that crying is often a sign that early signals have been missed.

AFTER CAESAREAN BIRTHS WITH AN EPIDURAL/SPINAL

Skin-to-skin contact between mother and baby should begin as soon as they are able and usually starting on the delivery table.

AFTER CAESAREAN BIRTHS UNDER GENERAL ANAESTHESIA

Skin-to-skin contact should commence within 30 min of the mother being able to respond.

IF A BABY NEEDS RESUSCITATION

Following effective resuscitation, the baby may be given to the mother at any stage, unwrapped and placed in skin-to-skin contact.

FOR INFANTS AT RISK OF HYPOGLYCAEMIA

Providing both mother and baby are well, infants should have skin-to-skin contact and an early feed on the labour ward (e.g. a breastfeed, expressed breast milk or formula). If the baby is otherwise well, blood glucose measurement before 3 h is not clinically helpful and may disrupt the first contact between mother and baby, and interfere with early feeding.

IF THE INFANT IS TRANSFERRED TO THE NEONATAL UNIT

If skin-to-skin contact and the initiation of breastfeeding is unavoidably delayed, a woman should be reassured that having uninterrupted skin-to-skin contact at a later stage may be of equal benefit. She should also be reassured that she will be shown how to hand express her milk and maintain lactation until her baby is able to feed.

MOTHERS WITH SPECIAL CIRCUMSTANCES

Even in the rare situation of a mother being transferred to an intensive care unit, effective support for establishing lactation is possible.

REFERENCES

1. Salariya EM, Easton PM, Cater JI. Duration of breast-feeding after early initiation and frequent feeding. *Lancet* 1978;II:1141–3

2. Widstrom AM, Wahlberg V, Matthiesen AS, *et al*. Short-term effects of early suckling and touch of the nipple on maternal behaviour. *Early Hum Develop* 1990;21:153–63
3. Van den Bosch CA, Bullough CH. Effect of early suckling on term neonates' core body temperature. *Ann Trop Paediatr* 1990;10:347–53
4. Christensson K, Siles C, Moreno L, *et al*. Temperature, metabolic adaptation and crying in healthy full-term newborns cared for skin-to-skin or in a cot. *Acta Paediatr* 1992;81:488–93
5. Righard L, Alade MO. Effect of delivery room routines on success of first breastfeed. *Lancet* 1990;336:1105–7
6. Widstrom AM, Ransjo-Arvidson AB, Christensson K, Matthiesen AS, Winberg J, Urnas-Moberg K. Gastric suction in healthy newborn infants. Effects on circulation and developing feeding behaviour. *Acta Paediatr* 1987;76:566–72
7. Rajan L. The impact of obstetric procedures and analgesia/anaesthesia during labour and delivery on breast feeding. *Midwifery* 1994;10:87–103
8. Nissen E, Lilja G, Matthiesen AS, Ransjo-Arvidsson AB, Uvnas-Moberg K, Widstrom AM. Effects of maternal pethidine on infants' developing breast-feeding behaviour. *Acta Paediatr* 1995;84:140–5
9. Renfrew MJ, *et al*. Enabling women to breastfeed: a review of practices which promote or inhibit breastfeeding – with evidence-based guidance for practice. Leeds, UK: University of Leeds, 1998
10. Righard L, Alade MO. Sucking technique and its effect on success of breast-feeding. *Birth* 1992;19:185–9
11. Widstrom AM, Thingstrom-Paulsson J. The position of the tongue during rooting reflexes elicited in newborn infants before the first suckle. *Acta Paediatr* 1993;82:281–3

BIBLIOGRAPHY

Daly SEJ, *et al*. The determination of short-term breast volume changes and the rate of synthesis of human milk using computerised breast measurement. *Exp Physiol* 1992;77:79–87

Dodds R, Newburn M. Low blood glucose: an NCT investigation. *Modern Midwife* 1996;6:14–17

Fisher C, Inch S. Nipple confusion – who is confused? *J Pediatr* 1996;129:174

Foster K, et al. Infant Feeding 1995 ONS. London: The Stationary Office, 1997

Hawdon J, Ward Platt MP, Aynsley-Green A. Patterns of metabolic adaptation for term and preterm infants in the first neonatal week. *Arch Dis Child* 1992;67:657–65

Host A, Husby S, Gjesing B, Larsen JN, Lowenstein H. Prospective estimation of IgG, IgG subclass and IgE antibodies to dietary proteins in infants with cow milk allergy. Levels of antibodies to whole milk protein, BLG and oval-bumin in relation to repeated milk challenge and clinical course of cow milk allergy. *Allergy* 1992;47:218–29

Houston MJ, Howie PW, McNeilly AS. Factors affecting the duration of breastfeeding: 1. Measurement of breast milk intake in the first week of life. *Early Hum Develop* 1983;8:55–63

Neifert M, Seacat JM. Lactation insufficiency: a rational approach. *Birth* 1987;14:182–8

Neifert M, Lawrence R, Seacat J. Nipple confusion: toward a formal definition. *J Pediatr* 1995;126:s125–9

WHO Division of Child Health and Development. *Evidence for the Ten Steps to Successful Breastfeeding*. Geneva: WHO, 1998

Williams A. *Hypoglycaemia of the Newborn: Review of the Literature*. Geneva: WHO, 1997

10

The prevention of thromboembolism

INTRODUCTION

Along with hypertension in pregnancy, thromboembolism presents the greatest threat to the life of the pregnant woman. Admission to hospital is generally not for promoting bed rest, which in any case is not an effective cure for many conditions. Women who do spend periods immobile should be instructed on regular leg exercises. Maintaining mobility and early mobility after delivery is desirable.

At Caesarean section (CS), pneumatic boots should always be used. Thromboembolism stockings are also appropriate before delivery and afterwards for women at risk.

The low molecular weight heparin (LMWH), dalteparin, has replaced unfractionated heparin (UFH) as the treatment of choice for this indication within many UK institutions. LMWH has been found to be at least as effective as UFH in the thromboprophylaxis of surgical patients. In some incidences they may be superior to UFH.

Women identified as 'at risk' during the antenatal period should have a plan for labour written in their notes.

PROPHYLAXIS AGAINST THROMBOEMBOLIC DISEASE FOLLOWING CAESAREAN SECTION

At CS, pneumatic boots should always be used. A risk assessment profile of all patients undergoing elective or emergency CS should also be performed. Patients undergoing elective CS with uncomplicated pregnancy and no other factors require early mobilization and attention to hydration. Patients assessed as of moderate or high risk should all receive subcutaneous heparin and use thromboembolism stockings. Prophylaxis until the fifth postoperative day is advised (or until fully mobilized if longer). The use of subcutaneous heparin as thromboprophylaxis in patients with an epidural or spinal block remains contentious. Current evidence from general and orthopaedic surgery does not point to an increased risk of spinal haematoma. The risk of deep vein thrombosis (DVT) or pulmonary embolism in pregnant patients undergoing CS seems to be greater.

PROPHYLAXIS AGAINST THROMBOEMBOLISM IN PREGNANCY

Patients with a previous history of venous thromboembolism in pregnancy/puerperium and no other known thrombotic risk factor should receive thromboprophylaxis for up to 6 weeks postpartum (subcutaneous heparin and then oral warfarin if desired). History of previous thromboembolism outside of pregnancy and puerperium does not increase the risk antenatally. Patients at high risk (e.g. those having had multiple episodes of thromboembolism) may require heparin throughout pregnancy.

DIAGNOSIS AND MANAGEMENT OF DEEP VEIN THROMBOSIS IN PREGNANCY AND PUERPERIUM

The importance of accurate diagnosis of DVT in pregnancy cannot be overstressed. Inappropriate full anticoagulation carries risks to the mother and fetus and has long-term implications regarding future contraceptive methods and management in subsequent pregnancy. Real-time ultrasound scanning combined with pulsed Doppler or colour flow Doppler being non-invasive and with a high degree of specificity and sensitivity are the first choice first-line diagnostic techniques for DVT in pregnancy. If ultrasound is inconclusive, then limited venography can be performed in the second and third trimester, with appropriate shielding of the fetus, to confirm the diagnosis.

The duration of anticoagulation in patients with proven DVT should be discussed with the haematologists, but likely to be for a minimum of 3 months.

There is no contraindication to breastfeeding when the woman is taking either heparin or warfarin.

TABLE 10-1. RISK ASSESSMENT PROFILE FOR THROMBOEMBOLISM IN CAESAREAN SECTION

LOW RISK – Early mobilization, hydration and leg stockings
Elective Caesarean section – uncomplicated pregnancy and no other risk factors

MODERATE RISK – Heparin prophylaxis and leg stockings
- Age > 35 years
- Obesity (> 80 kg)
- Para 4 or more
- Gross varicose veins
- Current infection
- Pre-eclampsia
- Immobility prior to surgery (> 4 days)
- Major current illness, e.g. heart or lung disease cancer, inflammatory bowel disease, nephrotic syndrome
- Emergency Caesarean section in labour

Dalteparin
Subcutaneous 2500 IU 1–2 h before surgery, then subcutaneous 2500 IU each day

HIGH RISK – Heparin prophylaxis and leg stockings
- A patient with three or more moderate risk factors from above
- Extended major pelvic or abdominal surgery, e.g. Caesarean hysterectomy
- Patients with a personal or family history of deep vein thrombosis, pulmonary embolism or thrombophilia, paralysis of lower limbs.
- Patients with antiphospholipid antibody (cardiolipin antibody or lupus anticoagulant)

Dalteparin
Subcutaneous 2500 IU 1–2 h before surgery, then subcutaneous 2500 IU 8–12 h postsurgery, then 5000 IU each day thereafter or subcutaneous 5000 IU on the evening before surgery, then, subcutaneous 5000 IU each day postsurgery

BIBLIOGRAPHY

Clements RV. *Safe Practice in Obstetrics and Gynaecology*. Edinburgh: Churchill de Swiet M, ed. Medical Disorders in Obstetric Practice, Fourth edition. Oxford: Blackwell Science, 1995:683

Edmonds DK, ed. *Dewhurst's Textbook of Obstetrics and Gynaecology for Postgraduates*, Sixth edition. Oxford: Blackwell Science, 1999:622

James DK, *et al. High Risk Pregnancy*. London: WB Saunders, 1994:1318

11

Induction, stimulation and augmentation of labour

DEFINITIONS

Induction is the process of starting labour artificially. Stimulation is the process of inducing contractions following rupture of membranes. Augmentation is the correction of inefficient uterine action once labour has started.

INDUCTION

Preparation

Most women are admitted early on the morning of induction. Whether the woman is an inpatient or has been admitted that day, the senior house officer should check the period of gestation and confirm the indication for induction. Part of the decision to induce will have been cervical assessment. The consultant under whom the woman is booked should be made aware of any elective inductions of labour for any indication other than postmaturity.

Under some circumstances induction of labour (IOL) will not be possible at the anticipated time. Women for induction should be informed on the morning of the induction by a member of the labour team that they can come in. If the induction is delayed, the mother should be informed as soon as possible.

The doctor and midwives caring for the woman should ensure that she and her partner, if appropriate, understand and agree with the planned procedure. It is important to remember that women who had hoped for an uncomplicated labour may be extremely disappointed when the need for induction becomes clear. Staff should try to minimize this disappointment by ensuring that the woman remains fully involved in decisions regarding all aspects of her care. Use of prostaglandin does not always result in the onset of labour, and it is important that this is explained to the woman before it is administered. A primigravida woman with an unfavourable cervix (and her partner) should be warned of a possibly lengthy process.

TABLE 11-1. MODIFIED BISHOP'S SCORE (CALDER SCORE)

When labour is being induced or patients with premature membrane rupture are being stimulated it is important to score the cervix. The maximum score is 10

Score	0	1	2
Dilatation of cervix (cm)	< 1	1–2	2–4
Effacement of cervix	> 4 cm long	2–4 cm long	1–2 cm long
Consistency	hard/firm	soft/average	soft and stretchable
Position	posterior	mid	anterior
Station	3 cm above ischial spines	2 cm above ischial spines	At ischial spines

METHODS OF INDUCTION OF LABOUR

The method chosen for induction will be influenced by several factors including: the period of gestation, the indication for induction, any underlying medical/obstetric problems and the favourability of the cervix. The most commonly used methods are: prostaglandin vaginal gel, artificial rupture of the membranes (ARM) and ARM/oxytocin infusion (if needed).

The method and need for IOL of a woman with a uterine scar (e.g. previous Caesarean section [CS] or uterine surgery) should have been discussed with the relevant consultant. If this has not occurred it should be discussed with the relevant consultant or the consultant on call. No more than one dose of prostaglandin should be given to a woman with a uterine scar unless discussed with the consultant on call.

PROSTAGLANDIN VAGINAL GEL

Prostaglandins should be used in preference to oxytocin when IOL is undertaken in most circumstances. Women with an uncomplicated pregnancy who require IOL (e.g. for postmaturity, rupture of membranes without evidence of infection) may be admitted to the ante-natal ward. Women with a complicated pregnancy (e.g. intrauterine growth retardation, maternal illness, grande multiparity, previous CS, reduced liquor not due to rupture of membranes) should be induced on the labour ward. Multiparity alone is not a reason for IOL on the labour ward.

For women of low risk, the first dose of prostaglandin may be prescribed the night prior to IOL or in the antenatal clinic. The dose of prostaglandin gel will depend on the parity of the woman, the degree of uterine activity and the state of her cervix. Prostaglandin gel should not be used in a woman who is contracting unless discussed with the senior specialist registrar or consultant on-call.

The fetal heart is monitored prior to insertion of the gel for 20–30 mins. After this first administration of gel, the woman is encouraged to mobilize if she wishes. The fetal heart should be monitored prior to each gel insertion and with the onset of contractions after each gel. Women should be encouraged to report the onset of contractions to their midwife. After 4–6 h a second vaginal examination is performed, and if no significant contractions are occurring then a second gel is inserted. If contractions have occurred, but the cervix has not changed signifi-cantly, then prostagladin E_2 1 mg is given.

TABLE 11-2. DOSE OF PROSTAGLANDIN REQUIRED IN PRIMIPAROUS AND MULTIPAROUS WOMEN

Primiparous women	
Cervical score	**Dose**
< 5	2 mg prostaglandin gel
5–7	1 mg prostaglandin gel
> 7 + 2–3 cm dilated	ARM
Multiparous women	
Cervical score	**Dose**
< 5	1 mg prostaglandin gel
5–7	1 mg prostaglandin gel
> 7 + 2–3 cm dilated	ARM

If after any of the gel insertions labour becomes established, then ARM and subsequent oxytocin infusion may be appropriate. Care must be taken not to superimpose the oxytocic effect of ARM and oxytocin too soon after prostaglandin application, as this may hyperstimulate the uterus and lead to fetal compromise. While great caution should be exercised in giving prostaglandin to women with contractions to avoid uterine hyperstimulation, occasional painless tightenings do not constitute significant uterine activity and are not a contraindication to the administration of prostaglandins. Sytocinon should not be used within 4 h of the last prostaglandin gel. In low-risk women, intermittent monitoring may be used after 10 h on prostaglandins (see page 23). Continuous electronic fetal monitoring must be recommenced if there is any suspicion of uterine hyperstimulation.

ARTIFICIAL RUPTURE OF MEMBRANES ALONE

This option is normally reserved for multiparous women with a favourable cervix (≥ 2–3 cm dilatation) and an engaged head. An abdominal palpation should be performed to confirm the presentation and engagement of the presenting part. Providing that these are satisfactory, a vaginal examination is then performed and the membranes ruptured using an amnihook. If, on vaginal examination, the presenting part is high, the decision to rupture the membranes will need to be reconsidered. If labour is not established 2–4 h after the ARM, a syntocinon infusion should be commenced.

ARTIFICIAL RUPTURE OF MEMBRANES AND OXYTOCIN INFUSION

Following the ARM a 20 min trace of the fetal heart is recorded and, provided that this is satisfactory, an oxytocin infusion is commenced.

PROLONGED INDUCTION OF LABOUR

If, in the evening of the induction, labour has not been established, then the specialist registrar should review the situation and, after consultation with the woman and her partner, decide which of the following should occur:

- rest overnight and a third dose of prostaglandin gel given at 06:00, unless labour is already established

- rest for 24 h and restart induction the following day or

- ARM and an oxytocin infusion commenced

If labour has not been established after a second day of attempted induction, the senior specialist registrar or consultant should review the situation and after consultation with the woman and her partner decide which of the following should occur:

- the membranes are ruptured and an oxytocin infusion commenced

- rest for 24 h and restart induction the next day or

- perform CS

STIMULATION OF LABOUR

Labour is usually stimulated in term pregnancy when the membranes have been ruptured for more than 24–96 h, contractions have not commenced and delivery is desired. The exact time of induction within this period may be chosen at the convenience of the woman. Up to this time, the woman should check her temperature two to four times a day and have the fetal heart rate (FHR) checked either at home or in hospital. A fetal assessment unit/ultrasound scan assessment is not necessary in uncomplicated cases. A low vaginal swab should be taken and the culture result reviewed at 24–48 h. If the culture is positive for group B streptococcal infection, this should be treated and stimulation of labour recommenced (see chapter 16). If a woman wishes expectant management for > 96 h, she should be reviewed by the relevant senior specialist registrar or consultant.

In cases of previous CS or breech presentation, the senior specialist registrar or consultant must be consulted. Prolonged oxytocic therapy in cases with a previous CS scar is problematic. If there is lack of satisfactory progress of cervical dilatation over a 2-h period in such women the senior specialist registrar should be consulted and a CS should be considered. The risk of cord prolapse in a breech presentation should always be considered.

The method used to stimulate labour will be either an oxytocin infusion or prostaglandin gel depending on the circumstances and wishes of the woman and the relevant consultant. In some cases, the forewaters will not have broken and this should be performed. In a parous woman, a good stretch of the cervix will also contribute to the process continuing. The exact method of stimulation will usually be determined by cervical score, parity and the views of the woman.

AUGMENTATION OF LABOUR

Augmentation is normally considered if labour progresses at a rate of a 0.5 cm/h or less. ARM should first be performed and the vaginal examination repeated 2 h later. If, after 2 h, normal progress of labour has not resumed, syntocinon is normally commenced after exclusion of obvious obstructive forms of delay . If no significant dilatation of the cervix has occurred over a 4 h period in a labouring woman and augmentation of labour is declined by the woman, the senior specialist registrar or consultant on call must be informed.

RELATIVE CONTRAINDICATIONS TO SYNTOCINON

Before starting syntocinon, review and examination (vaginal and abdominal) by an specialist registrar and discussion with the senior specialist registrar is needed for cases of malpresentation, previous CS or multiparity. Before starting syntocinon, prior review by an specialist registrar is needed for: any abnormality of the cardiotocograph or maternal cardiac disease (use syringe pump).

MONITORING IN INDUCED, STIMULATED AND AUGMENTED LABOURS

In these circumstances it is considered normal practice to monitor both the FHR and uterine contractions continuously. This should not be a reason to restrict a woman's mobility. If continuous electronic fetal monitoring is declined the senior specialist registrar should be informed. As an alternative, the FHR should be measured ultrasonically after every contraction. The exact FHR and any abnormalities should be recorded in the notes after each recording.

REGIMEN FOR SYNTOCINON INFUSION

Syntocinon is normally added to normal saline. The normal starting concentrations are 8 U/l for primigravida women and 4 U/l for multiparous women. Syntocinon should be administered using a syringe pump after one bag of syntocinon has been used. It is not normally necessary to give any other fluids intravenously unless medically indicated or an epidural is required.

Escalation of the tabulated dose at 15-min intervals permits the optimum dose to be reached in a reasonable period of time by titration against contractions. Contractions should not be more than four in 10 min and should not last longer than 60 s. The uterus should relax adequately between contractions. Effective uterine activity can normally be achieved at 12 mU/min. Syntocinon should not be used at a rate greater than 24 mU/min unless discussed with the senior specialist registrar. Particular care to exclude uterine hyperstimulation or fetal distress should be taken when using dosages of syntocinon over 8 mU/min.

TABLE 11-3. OXYTOCIN DOSE CALCULATION (mU/min)

Time (min)	ml/h	Multigravid women (4 U/l)	Primigravid women (8 U/l)
0	30	2	4
15	60	4	8
30	90	6	12
45	120	8	16
60	150	10	20
75	180	12	24

SIDE-EFFECTS OF SYNTOCINON INFUSION

If any of the following occur stop the infusion and seek medical advice:

- Fetal bradycardia or other abnormality
- Uterine hypertony or
- Breathlessness (beware pulmonary oedema and/or hyponatraemia)

UTERINE HYPERCONTRACTILITY WITH INDUCTION AGENTS

Should uterine hypercontractility occur with induction agents, the following should be done:

- Stop syntocinon infusion
- Give subcutaneous terbutaline 0.25 mg if uterine hypercontractility associated with prostaglandin and
- Consider delivery within 30 min if suspected or confirmed fetal compromise

CARE FOLLOWING DELIVERY

Following delivery the intravenous oxytocin should be continued at the same rate for 1 h. In cases where labour has been particularly prolonged with oxytocic use then high-dose (10 IU/h) oxytocin therapy should be given for 2 h and then discontinued. By preference this should be given via a syringe pump. This also applies to CS when syntocinon has been used during labour.

BIBLIOGRAPHY

Clements RV. *Safe Practice in Obstetrics and Gynaecology.* Edinburgh: Churchill Livingstone, 1994:492

Edmonds DK, ed. *Dewhurst's Textbook of Obstetrics and Gynaecology for Postgraduates,* Sixth edition. Oxford: Blackwell Science, 1999:622

Induction of Labour: RCOG Evidence-Based Guidelines Number 9. London: RCOG Press, 2001

James DK, et al. *High-Risk Pregnancy.* London: WB Saunders, 1994:1318

12

Caesarean section

Women are encouraged to consider having Caesarean section (CS) under spinal and/or epidural anaesthesia rather than general anaesthesia, especially if it is an elective procedure.

The operating surgeon must see the patient and discuss the nature of the operation and respond to any questions or requests prior to the patient being taken into theatre. The same person should aim to review the woman and discuss the events around the delivery within 2 days of any unplanned CS.

The specialist registrar should be scrubbed in theatre for all lower segment CS (LSCS) procedures. If the specialist registrar is unavailable the senior specialist registrar should be present and scrubbed.

If the LSCS is being performed for placenta praevia the senior specialist registrar must be present in theatre. The consultant on call should be made aware prior to any LSCS for placenta praevia.

For anterior placenta praevia or placenta praevia in the presence of a previous LSCS, the consultant should be in theatre.

The indication for CS must always be clearly stated and documented in the notes by the member of staff taking that decision. All elective CS decisions must be discussed with the woman's consultant. All emergency CS decisions must be discussed with the consultant on call unless the decision has been foreseen and discussed within 2 h.

ANTACID THERAPY

Emergency LSCS

When the decision is made to perform an LSCS, the following drugs should normally be given in the delivery room: intravenous ranitidine 50 mg and intravenous metoclopramide 10 mg. When the woman arrives in the anaesthetic room, she should be given sodium citrate 30 ml orally.

ELECTIVE LSCS

Most women scheduled to have an elective CS come in to hospital on the morning of the operation. All relevant documentation must be made available to the woman upon the her admission. This documentation should include consent forms, ranitidine prescriptions and other administrative documents.

In-patients on the evening prior to the operation should be reviewed and given oral ranitidine 150 mg and oral metoclopramide 10 mg. Additionally ranitidine 150 mg and oral metoclopramide 10 mg should be given at least 1 h prior to the administration of the anaesthetic.

FOR WOMEN AT HIGH RISK OF CAESAREAN SECTION IN LABOUR

During the course of labour women at high risk of CS should be given oral ranitidine 150 mg and metoclopramide 10 mg every 8 h. If these drugs cannot be administered orally they should be given intravenously. The woman should also be prepared for theatre using a checklist.

Infection control

It has been reported that at least 10% of latex gloves have small perforations. Double gloves should be worn to avoid transmission of blood-borne viruses for all CS procedures, regardless of known blood-borne virus status.

In most circumstances blunt needles should be used for all internal layers. If clips are not used for skin closure, sharp needles can be used.

All women having either elective or emergency CS are given cefuroxime 750 mg and metronidazole 500 mg, unless specifically contraindicated. It is appropriate as a routine to mention both the use of an oxytocic (usually syntocinon 10 U IV) and the antibiotic to the anaesthetist at this time.

TABLE 12-1. POST-CAESAREAN SECTION ANALGESIA

Drug and dosage	Notes
Diclofenac 100 mg per rectum at the end of the surgical procedure	Contraindications: known impairment of renal function, platelet count < 80 000, history of allergic reaction to NSAIDs
Diclofenac 75 mg oral by regular prescription every 12 h	Contraindications as above. Note that the first oral dose should be at least 8 h after the rectal diclofenac given in theatre
Morphine sulphate 10–15 mg intramuscular as required	Maximum frequency every 3 h
Paracetamol 1 g regularly 6-hourly	Maximum frequency every 6 h
Metoclopramide 10 mg oral/intramuscular as required	Maximum frequency every 6 h
Ondansetron 4 mg intramuscular /intravenous as required	Maximum frequency every 6 h. To be prescribed only if metoclopramide is ineffective for antiemetic therapy

THE RESPONSIBILITY AND ROLE OF THE MIDWIFE IN THEATRE

Responsibility

The midwife is responsible for the provision of care to the mother and baby pre- and postoperatively, including the documentation. The midwife has a responsibility to promote and provide continuity of care, a safe environment and ensure that the psychological and physical needs of the mother and baby are met. The midwife should undertake the responsibility for the preparation of the mother preoperatively, take the baby in theatre and provide postoperative care for them both. In the event of a general anaesthetic, she should remain with the mother until she is anaesthetized.

The midwife's role

Preoperatively, the midwife must:

- Confirm that the woman understands the reason for the operation (e.g. CS and what it involves)

- Check that the consent form is signed and the preoperative checklist is completed

- Escort the mother to the anaesthetic room, once the woman is prepared for theatre
- Auscultate the fetal heart and ensure cardiotocography monitoring is undertaken when appropriate
- Ensure that the resuscitation/cot/incubator equipment are ready for use
- Ensure the paediatrician and neonatal unit are informed prior to the operation if there is a possibility that the baby will be transferred there
- Hand over the care of the woman to the theatre team and anaesthetist for the insertion of the epidural (however, the midwife will remain with the woman if so requested)
- Ensure that once the epidural is effective or the woman is anaesthetized, the bladder is catherized
- Ensure that the paediatrician is called to attend the delivery and
- Organize that a porter is requested to bring a bed from the postnatal ward

Perioperatively, the midwife must be ready to assist in neonatal care and must:

- Ensure that he/she is scrubbed-up ready for taking the baby
- Assist the paediatrician with resuscitation of the baby (if necessary) and
- Promote family contact for mothers having epidural anaesthesia

Prior to leaving theatre with mother and baby, the midwife must:

- Check placenta and membranes, taking cord blood for cord pH and Coombs' test (if required)
- Send the placenta for histology examination if the baby is to be sent to the neonatal unit, otherwise dispose of placenta in placenta bins
- Clean and restock resuscitaire and
- Examine and weigh baby, giving care as with normal practice

In recovery, the woman should be under continuous clinical observation for at least 30 min until discharged from the recovery area. During the recovery period the woman will be cared for by the theatre team. Once the woman is conscious and her observations stable, the care will then be handed back to the midwife.

Whilst the patient is in the recovery area (outside anaesthetic room), a midwife or a labour ward nurse will be in attendance. For each bed there must be an oxygen outlet and breathing system for 100% oxygen, electrical sockets, pulse oximeter, electrocardiography monitor, suction unit, blood pressure meter and easily available disposables (IV cannulas, giving sets etc.). The recovery area must have a defibrillator, emergency drug box and emergency buzzer. All staff looking after recovering patients must have training in recovery care and in cardiopulmonary resuscitation.

The midwife must ensure that the patient's vital signs are monitored and documented in accordance with her condition. The following observations must be documented on a suitable chart at least every 15 min (every 5 min for the first 15 min): oxygen saturation, respiratory rate, heart rate and rhythm, blood pressure, blood loss from wound, vagina, and drain, and check that the intravenous infusion is running correctly. The mother and baby may be moved to another room to await transfer to the ward, but they should always have a person with them during this time. Finally, the midwife needs to inform the postnatal ward prior to transfer and accompany the woman and baby to the postnatal ward.

DOCUMENTATION

The midwife should complete the following:

* Mother's/baby's notes, including observation charts
* Computer data and
* Birth register

BIBLIOGRAPHY

Clements RV. *Safe Practice in Obstetrics and Gynaecology.* Edinburgh: Churchill Livingstone, 1994:492

Edmonds DK, ed. *Dewhurst's Textbook of Obstetrics and Gynaecology for Postgraduates,* Sixth edition. Oxford: Blackwell Science, 1999:622

13

Vaginal instrumental deliveries

All women undergoing an instrumental delivery must be catheterized and have adequate analgesia. The specialist registrar will be informed and be present in the room for all forceps and ventouse deliveries.

The position of the baby's head should be checked by the specialist registrar before application of the forceps/ventouse. If the junior specialist registrar is unavailable the senior specialist registrar must be present in the delivery room.

All forceps deliveries other than occipito anterior (OA) below the ischial spines should be performed in theatre, unless the specialist registrar considers that the delivery should be straightforward. The senior specialist registrar must be present and clinically assess all forceps/ventouse deliveries undertaken in theatre. Anaesthetic and theatre staff should be present and informed consent for a Caesarean section (CS) procedure should be obtained prior to attempted vaginal delivery.

If trial of instrumental delivery fails and a CS is needed, then the CS should be performed by either the senior specialist registrar or the junior specialist registrar and both should be present.

In all babies who have passed meconium, the oropharnx should be sucked out as soon as possible (e.g. at the perineum). However, if the baby needs urgent paediatric aid then the baby should be passed to the attendant paediatricians as soon as possible and this should not be delayed by attempts to suck out the oropharnx.

Keeping good notes is as important for vaginal instrumental as it is for CS. It is recommended that an operation note form or the instrumental delivery page of the obstetric notes is used.

For ventouse delivery, the number of pulls and the total cup application time should be recorded. These should not exceed three pulls and 20 min respectively unless delivery is very imminent.

For forceps delivery, the ease (or otherwise) of application, position of the fetal head, number of pulls and the degree of traction should be recorded. Forceps should only be applied after attempted ventouse if there has been unexpected total equipment failure of the ventouse or if the ventouse cup has slipped from the fetal head when the head is in the OA or occipito posterior position and is nearly crowning.

Cord arterial and venous samples should be taken for blood gases in all cases

BIBLIOGRAPHY

Clements RV. *Safe Practice in Obstetrics and Gynaecology*. Edinburgh: Churchill Livingstone, 1994:492

Edmonds DK, ed. *Dewhurst's Textbook of Obstetrics and Gynaecology for Postgraduates*, Sixth edition. Oxford: Blackwell Science, 1999:622

James DK, *et al*. High Risk Pregnancy. London: WB Saunders, 1994:1318

14

Cardiotocograph interpretation and fetal blood sampling

The name, date and time should always be checked when reviewing a cardiotocograph (CTG) trace. If at all uncertain about the interpretation of a CTG trace, staff should always seek a more senior opinion.

TABLE 14-1. DEFINITIONS OF CARDIOTOCOGRAPHY TERMS

Bradycardia
Baseline heart rate of less than 110 beats/min
Tachycardia
Baseline heart rate greater than 160 beats/min
Baseline variability
The variation of the base line over a particular band width
Normal   > 5 beats/min
Abnormal   0–5 beats/min
Accelerations
A transient heart rate increase of 15 beats/min or more lasting 15 s or more

(continued)

TABLE 14-1. (continued)

Decelerations
A transient decrease in heart rate of more than 15 beats/min and lasting 15 s
or more
Early decelerations
Onset with contractions and recovering within contractions. Less than 40
beats/min drop from baseline
Late decelerations
Onset and recovery out of phase with contraction
Variable deceleration
Decelerations that do not have a consistent relationship in time or frequency
with contractions
A reactive trace
The recording of at least 2 accelerations in a 20-min period

TABLE 14-2. CLASSIFICATION OF FETAL HEART RATE PATTERN COMPONENTS

Reassuring characteristics
Baseline 110–160
Variability > 5 beats/min
No decelerations
Accelerations present

Non-reassuring characteristics
Baseline 100–109 or 161–180
Variability < 5 beats/min for 40–90 min
Early decelerations
Variable decelerations
Single prolonged deceleration for up to 3 min

Abnormal characteristics
Baseline < 100 or > 180
Variability < 5 beats/min for > 90 min
Atypical variable decelerations
Late decelerations
Single prolonged deceleration for > 3 min

TABLE 14-3. CLASSIFICATION OF A CARDIOTOCOGRAPH

Normal

All four features fall into the reassuring category, e.g.:
Normal baseline
Normal variability
Accelerative pattern and
Moderate bradycardia (110–120) with normal variability

Suspicious

A cardiotocograph in which one feature falls into the non-reassuring category, but the remainder are reassuring, e.g.:
Moderate tachycardia (150–170) with normal variability or
Moderate bradycardia (100–110) with normal variability

Pathological

A cardiotocograph in which two or more features fall into the non-reassuring category or one or more features fall into the abnormal category, e.g.:
Moderate tachycardia (150–170) with reduced variability
Prolonged bradycardia for longer than 3 min
Late decelerations and
Severe variable decelerations

FETAL BLOOD SAMPLING

The use of fetal blood sampling (FBS) reduces the known increase in Caesarean section rate that is associated with continuous fetal heart rate monitoring.

Indications for fetal blood sampling
FBS should be considered in the following cases: an abnormal trace (suspicious or pathological) that continues for more than 30 min in the (> 34 weeks) normally grown baby or for more than 10 min in a growth restricted and/or preterm baby; the appearance of meconium staining for the first time during labour in conjunction with a suspicious trace; or rotation delivery is planned and the CTG is not normal.

When not to perform fetal blood sampling
FBS should not be attempted in the following cases:

• If the clinical picture demands early delivery

- When a severly abnormal trace prompts immediate delivery

- When the CTG changes are due to oxytocic overstimulation and resolve when oxytocinon is stopped

- When there is associated persistent failure to progress in labour

- During or soon after an episode of prolonged bradycardia

- If spontaneous vaginal delivery is imminent or easy instrumental vaginal delivery is possible

- In a case of trial of scar (it is not known whether FBS results in such women predict fetal outcome or uterine scar dehiscence)

- In women with proven chorioamnionitis (non-reassuring CTG abnormalities indicate delivery; a FBS result may be falsely reassuring) or

- In women who are HIV- or hepatitis B-positive, or in women whom the baby may have thrombocytopaenia or bleeding disorder

NORMAL BLOOD GAS AND PH VALUES

Normal blood gas and pH values are as follows: pH > 7.3, PO_2 > 20 mmHg (> 2.6 kPa), PCO_2 < 50 mmHg (< 8 kPa) and base excess > -8 mEq/l.

ACTION TO BE TAKEN

A pH of less than 7.2 indicates urgent delivery (within 30 min), while a pH of 7.2–7.25 indicates that the FBS should be repeated in 30 min regardless of the CTG. pH values of 7.25–7.3 are suspicious. The FBS should be repeated in 30–60 min if the trace continues to be abnormal, but need not be repeated if the trace becomes normal.

BIBLIOGRAPHY

Clements RV. *Safe Practice in Obstetrics and Gynaecology*. Edinburgh: Churchill Livingstone, 1994:492

Edmonds DK, ed. *Dewhurst's Textbook of Obstetrics and Gynaecology for Postgraduates*, Sixth edition. Oxford: Blackwell Science, 1999:622

James DK, et al. *High Risk Pregnancy*. London: WB Saunders, 1994:1318

The Use of Electronic Fetal Monitoring: the Use and Interpretation of Cardiotocography in Intrapartum Fetal Surveillance (Guideline no. 8). London: RCOG Press, 2001

15

Preterm labour

INTRODUCTION

With the facilities currently available the outcome for babies delivered at 32–37 weeks' gestation is extremely good and, for this reason, labour is normally allowed to proceed at this gestation. The guidelines that follow apply to a situation where labour occurs in a singleton pregnancy that is otherwise uncomplicated. If other complications exist, a senior specialist registrar or consultant's opinion must always be sought before the management plan is finalized. Neonatal morbidity and mortality is so low after 32 weeks' gestation that the measures described below relate in the main to idiopathic preterm labour prior to this gestation. The management suggestions below may also be followed at 32–35 weeks, except that tocolytics are less frequently used. After 35 weeks, *in utero* transfer, tocolyics and maternal steroids are rarely required.

DIAGNOSIS

A diagnosis of pre-term labour is made if painful contractions are occurring more frequently than one every 10 min and the dilatation and/or effacement of the cervix alters between examinations 2 h apart. The level of the presenting part and the presence or absence of fetal breathing movements may also be useful diagnostic tools. In practice, preterm labour is exceptionally difficult to diagnose and, as only 50% of women considered to be in preterm labour actually deliver within 48 h of the diagnosis, it is better considered as threatened preterm labour.

MANAGEMENT

On admission, the duty specialist registrar should be informed and he/she should assess the woman. A speculum examination of the cervix should be undertaken and a high vaginal swab taken. Following any necessary consultation, the proposed management plan should be explained and discussed with the woman and documented in the notes. The use of tocolytics must be discussed with the consultant on call. The plan of action will depend upon many factors. Care must be taken in multiple pregnancies. It is very helpful if a paediatrician is involved early in discussions with the parents concerning management.

MULTIPLE PREGNANCY

Women with a multiple pregnancy are at particular risk of cardiorespiratory complications as a result of the administration of beta-mimetics and steroids in the management of preterm labour. The risks are proportional to the number of babies. Particular care and detailed discussion is necessary with the consultant on call.

PRETERM RUPTURE OF THE MEMBRANES UNACCOMPANIED BY CONTRACTIONS

Women presenting with preterm, prelabour rupture of the membranes in the absence of contractions need to be seen as quickly as possible and a management plan agreed. The risk to the fetus in this situation is increased.

If less than 32 weeks gestation:

- The specialist registrar should be informed

- An aseptic speculum examination should be performed to confirm the diagnosis and examine the cervix

- A low vaginal swab should be obtained and sent for culture and sensitivity, and for the presence of chlamydial infection

- An ultrasound (US) scan may be performed to assess liquor volume, confirm presentation, confirm normality and estimate fetal weight

- The consultant on call should be informed

- A digital vaginal examination should not be performed

In the absence of any signs of infection, the aim would be to maintain the pregnancy until at least 34 weeks' gestation.
  If more than 32 weeks' gestation:

- An aseptic speculum examination should be performed to confirm the diagnosis and examine the cervix

- A low vaginal swab should be obtained and sent for culture and sensitivity, and for the presence of chlamydial infection

- An ultrasound scan should be performed to assess liquor volume, confirm presentation and estimate fetal weight and

- Further management should be discussed with the consultant, the woman and her partner

If the presentation is anything other than vertex, the risk of cord prolapse is increased. Conservative management under these circumstances must be discussed with a consultant.

As with preterm labour, it is essential to involve a paediatrician in the decision-making process. If possible the mother and her partner should be taken to the neonatal unit prior to the delivery where they can meet the medical and nursing staff and talk to them about the care that their baby may require.

MANAGEMENT OF DELIVERY OF THE PRETERM FETUS

Every case will need to be reviewed in detail when the mode of delivery is to be decided. As a general principle, if the presentation is abnormal and the baby is less than 34 weeks' gestation delivery will be by lower segment Caesarean section; if the presentation is cephalic, a vaginal delivery will be anticipated. Vaginal delivery should be conducted by a midwife and, if thought necessary, an episiotomy should be performed. A suitably qualified paediatrician and an experienced obstetric senior house officer or specialist registrar should always be present for the delivery. If assisted delivery is necessary, ventouse should not be used when the fetus is below 35 weeks' gestation. Every effort must be made to keep the parents fully informed and involved in these circumstances in order to minimize what may be an extremely stressful situation.

DELIVERIES OCCURRING BETWEEN 22 AND 26 WEEKS' GESTATION

On some occasions, labour will occur spontaneously at 22–26 weeks' gestation. In these instances the mother should always be seen by the specialist registrar and time taken to discuss with her how her labour is to be managed. It is essential for a paediatrician to be involved early in discussions with the parents concerning management. The fetal heart is generally not monitored in the first stage of labour if it has been decided that no action would be taken in the event of abnormalities being detected. Consideration should be given to monitoring the fetal heart in the second stage, as this may influence the way in which it is managed and it will be of importance to the neonatologist in considering resuscitation.

A suitably experienced paediatrician (senior specialist registrar or consultant) should be present at all such deliveries in case the baby is born alive and also to support the parents and examine the baby if the baby does not survive. The presence of a paediatrician at delivery does not imply that resuscitation will occur and this should have been made clear to the parents beforehand. It is essential, regardless of the period of gestation, that the baby is treated with the utmost respect and gentleness at birth and the wishes of the parents adhered to.

Women at gestations of between 16 and 23 weeks are generally managed on the maternity unit rather than the gynaecology ward.

GENERAL MEASURES IN THE ASSESSMENT OF THREATENED PRETERM LABOUR

Ensure that gestation is correctly estimated. If there is any doubt over menstrual dates, gestation must be checked against a first trimester (11–14 weeks) US scan, or failing this, the 23-week scan report. Otherwise, US dating on the labour ward is recommended, most accurately performed with reference to the BPD.

Analgesia should be given (unless delivery is imminent) as neccessary prior to examination, and the woman should be reassured.

Maternal pulse rate, blood pressure and hydration state should be recorded. Abdominal palpation is performed for presentation, uterine tenderness (degenerating fibroid, placental abruption or chorioamnionitis) and loin tenderness (urinary tract infection/pyelonephritis). Prior to 32 weeks, a specialist registrar should perform a speculum and/or digital examination. If there is a suspicion of prolonged premature rupture of membranes, a speculum examination should be performed in preference to a digital examination.

A portable US scan should be performed by the most experienced person present to determine: fetal heart(s), fetal movements, fetal lie, presentation, amniotic fluid index (AFI) (four-quadrant AFI in cm), placental position (if low, in relation to the internal cervical os), presence of retroplacental bleeding, fetal biometry (if unbooked), and cervical length and funnelling if the cervix is seen (usually the mother's bladder is partially filled to allow cervical visualization). Further management should include mid stream speciment urine (dip, and send for urgent microscopy); Venflon (14G) with full blood count (FBC), group and save serum, C-reactive protein; and low vaginal swab.

Depending on the clinical scenario, the following are management options:

- Maternal steroids should be given (two doses of intramuscular dexamethasone 12 mg 12 h apart) at the earliest opportunity. In the presence of type I diabetes mellitus, a sliding scale of insulin is required for 24 h from the first injection. A consultant opinion should be sought before starting steroid therapy on a woman with severe hypertension, diabetes mellitus or any signs of infection

- If a urinary tract infection is suspected, commence appropriate antibiotics (e.g. amoxycillin or a cephalosporin). However, most cases of preterm delivery are associated with intrauterine infection and therefore prophylaxis with intravenous penicillin 3 g stat then 1.5 g 4-hourly during labour (or 900 mg clindamycin 8-hourly if allergic to penicillin) should be given to the majority of women in preterm labour

- Rehydrate with crystalloid solution (e.g. Hartmann's solution)

- Analgesia as appropriate (co-proxamol orally or an intramuscular opiate). Opiates should be avoided if delivery is imminent. If they are given and delivery occurs soon after, the attendant paediatrician should be informed

- Depending on contraction frequency and fetal condition, continuous or intermittent cardiotocograph (CTG)

- Inform the consultant of admission, and liaise directly with the neonatal unit specialist registrar. If an *in utero* transfer is contemplated, then the consultant paediatrician will usually be contacted

- It is good practice for a request to be made for one of the paediatricians to introduce themselves to the woman and her partner (if there is time) to outline neonatal management and prognosis should delivery occur

- If labour is establishing, decide mode of delivery

- Where there are complicating factors (cervical suture, chorioamnionitis, multiple pregnancy) a consultant must be directly involved in the management of the preterm labour

- The mother must be told at the earliest opportunity whether she appears to be in established preterm labour or not, and whether an *in utero* transfer is likely to be required

- Tocolytics (see below)

TOCOLYICS

If the cervix is more than 3 cm dilated or the membranes are already ruptured, tocolytics are unlikely to be effective and would be used only in exceptional circumstances.

Tocolytics should only be given in threatened preterm labour prior to 32 weeks' gestation unless there are exceptional circumstances or prior to transfer. The preferred treatment at King's College Hospital is a glceryl trinitrate (GTN) patch. The second line treatment is intravenous ritodrine.

Do not use tocolytics if there is evidence of:

- Hypotension (less than 80 mmHg systolic or 50 mmHg diastolic pressure)

- Major fetal congenital abnormality, where tocolytics would not normally be used

- Fetal distress seen on the CTG

- Antepartum haemorrhage or history of recurrent vaginal bleeding

- Placenta praevia

- Cervical suture *in situ*

- Chorionamnionitis (pyrexia greater than 37.5°C with maternal tachycardia and uterine tenderness with or without offensive discharge per vaginam)

- Unexplained pyrexia

- Sensitivity or contraindication to nitrates or β-agonists

At the outset of treatment, monitoring of both maternal and fetal parameters should occur at least every 15 min. Once the condition of the patient on therapy is stable, monitoring may be undertaken every hour:

- abdominal examination to palpate contraction frequency and strength

- measurement of blood pressure, pulse and temperature and

- CTG trace recorded prior to and following GTN patch or ritodrine administration, followed by intermittent monitoring, provided that the screening CTG is normal and uterine contractions are settling

WOMEN GIVEN GTN

GTN has been shown in a multicentre study to reduce preterm delivery rate significantly compared to ritodrine or placebo[1] with minimal fetal or maternal effects[2] other than headache in 30% of women.

A GTN 10-mg/24-h patch is applied directly to the skin of the abdomen. If, following 1 h, there is no reduction in contraction frequency or strength then a second, additional patch is applied. The maximum number of patches that should be worn simultaneously is two. Mild headache is treated with paracetamol or co-proxamol. GTN patches remain in place for the full 24-h period, at the end of which they are removed and the patient re-assessed.

WOMEN GIVEN RITODRINE

β-agonists have been shown in a large multicentre study to reduce delivery within 24 and 48 h of treatment. The major side effects are chest pain, tremor, nausea and potentially fatal pulmonary oedema[3]

Ritodrine is given intravenously either via a syringe pump or via an Ivac or volumetric giving set. In the syringe pump protocol, ritodrine 90 mg is made up to 60 ml with 5% dextrose starting at an infusion rate of 1 ml/h (1.5 mg/h). This is increased by a further 1 ml after 15 min and thereafter at 2 ml increments every 15 min until the maternal pulse is greater than 120 or the contractions have ceased. In the Ivac/volumetric protocol, the dosage is 100 mg in 1000 ml 5% dextrose. The infusion commences at 5 drops/min or 15 ml/h (1.5 mg/h), is increased to 10 drops/min after 15 min and is then increased by 10 drops/min every 15 min until the maternal heart rate is 120 or the contractions have ceased.

Whilst the drug is in progress, the following observations must be performed:

- Maternal pulse is monitored continuously. Some electronic fetal heart rate monitors have the facility to do this. If a monitor is not available it should be checked every 15 min
- Blood-pressure should be checked every 15 min
- 4-Hourly BM stix
- Strict record of fluid balance must be kept
- 12-Hourly urea and electrolytes and blood glucose

Oral ritodrine is not used.

Ritodrine should be gradually reduced and discontinued 6 h after cessation of contractions.

CONTRAINDICATIONS TO BETA-MIMETICS

Beta-mimetics are usually contraindicated in any situation where the delivery is thought to be in the best interest of the mother and/or the baby. Table 1 presents conditions in which beta-mimetics may create such a situation and for this reason beta-mimetics should not be prescribed without further discussion with the consultant.

TABLE 15-1. CONDITIONS IN WHICH BETA-MIMETICS ARE CONTRAINDICATED

- Pre-existing cardiac disease
- Antepartum haemorrhage
- Diabetes
- Chorioamnionitis
- Severe hypertension
- Multiple pregnancy
- Intrauterine growth retardation

SIDE-EFFECTS OF BETA-MIMETICS

The side-effects of beta-mimetics include palpitations, chest discomfort, anxiety, sweating and tremor. Chest pain or dyspnoea should lead to the immediate cessation of the infusion.

REFERENCES

1. Lees CC, *et al*. Glyceryl trinitrate and ritodrine in tocolysis: an international multicenter randomized study. *Obstet Gynecol* 1999;94:403–8
2. Black RS, *et al*. Maternal and fetal cardiovascular effects of transdermal glyceryl trinitrate and intravenous ritodrine. Obstet Gynecol 1999;94:572–6
3. Canadian Preterm Labour Investigation Group. Treatment of preterm labor with the beta adrenergic agonist ritodrine. *N Engl J Med* 1992;327:308–12

BIBLIOGRAPHY

James DK, *et al*. *High Risk Pregnancy*. London: WB Saunders, 1994:1318

16

Prevention and treatment of neonatal group B streptococcal infection

Pregnant women found to have group B streptococcal (GBS) bacteruria at any stage antepartum should be offered treatment with oral penicillin four times a day for 10 days or erythromycin 500 mg four times a day if allergic to penicillin[1].

Further urine cultures should be sent to check for clearance of group B streptococcal infection 72 h following cessation of antibiotics. These women should also be offered intrapartum prophylaxis during labour whenever that supervenes.

Mothers who have ruptured membranes at term and are not in established labour should have a LVS performed. If they are still undelivered at 24–48 h, the culture results should be reviewed: if they are then known to be colonized with group B streptococcal infection then they should be treated immediately and stimulation of labour should be recommended[1-3].

Women with prolonged rupture of membranes in labour at any gestation should be treated 18 h after rupture of membranes.

Women with preterm rupture of membranes should be offered antibiotic treatment when they present, whether in labour or not.

Ideally, mothers with multiple pregnancy should be screened at 23 weeks of pregnancy and again at 34 weeks, and offered antibiotic prophylaxis during labour if they are found to be group B streptococcus carriers.

Mothers who were found to be group B streptococcus-positive at 23 weeks should be screened again at 34 weeks. If they go into premature labour and are known to be group B streptococcus-positive, antibiotic prophylaxis should be strongly recommended.

MATERNAL INTRAPARTUM PROPHYLAXIS

Intrapartum antibiotic prophylaxis with intravenous penicillin 3 g immediately then 1.5 g 4-hourly during labour (or 900 mg clindamycin 8-hourly if allergic to penicillin) should be used in the following circumstances, after sending a vaginal swab for culture[4-6]:

- Maternal pyrexia greater than 38°C for more than 1 h
- Delivery of a previous baby who developed neonatal group B streptococcal disease
- Women in labour with ruptured membranes for more than 18 h in whom the vaginal swab result is unknown
- Women in preterm labour (at < 37 weeks)
- Women who have been found on the selective screening programme to be carrying group B streptococcus vaginally in pregnancy (see above)
- Women who have had previous treatment for GBS bacteruria, as above

Alternative antibiotic regimens are ampicillin 1 g stat then 1 g 6-hourly or erythromycin 1 g 8-hourly for those who are allergic to penicillin.

MANAGEMENT OF NEWBORN INFANTS BORN TO MOTHERS GIVEN INTRAPARTUM PROPHYLAXIS.

Term babies (i.e. > 37 weeks of gestation) who are asymptomatic and whose mothers were treated more than 4 h prior to delivery need not be investigated or treated and can go to the postnatal ward. The respiratory rate and temperature should be taken 6-hourly for 24 h. These infants are not suitable for early discharge from the maternity hospital and should remain under observation for 48 h.

All term babies delivered to mothers who were given antibiotics less than 4 h before delivery, or whose mothers should have had antibiotics but did not, should have neonatal surface cultures, full blood count with a differential white cell count, C-reactive protein (CRP) and a blood culture sent. Surface cultures should be taken from the throat and the umbilicus. Gastric aspirate is not required. These babies should be treated whilst cultures are awaited.

Babies who are preterm (37 weeks or less) and asymptomatic and whose mothers had antibiotics at any stage of labour should have blood cultures, a full blood count and CRP performed in addition to surface surveillance cultures[7-11]. These babies should be treated with intravenous penicillin and gentamicin until the culture results are known. If the baby is well and otherwise suitable for transitional care then he or she may go to the postnatal ward with an intravenous cannula *in situ*. If symptoms are serious then a lumbar puncture should be done. A chest X-ray should be done if there are respiratory symptoms.

Symptomatic babies (pyrexia, tachypneoa, respiratory distress, lethargy) should be treated whenever they present at whatever gestation. Consideration should be given to performing a lumbar puncture in addition to the usual investigations[8-10].

Asymptomatic twin siblings of babies who develop group B streptococcal disease must be fully screened and treated with intravenous antibiotics. These babies have a 25-fold increased risk of group B streptococcal disease.

TREATMENT REGIMEN FOR NEONATES

The dose of penicillin should be 100 mg/kg/dose 12-hourly. The dose of gentamicin should be tailored to gestation and weight as given in the Neonatal Unit pharmacopeia. The course of antibiotics should be at least 10 days if blood cultures are positive and 14 days for proven meningitis. Antibiotics can be stopped after 48 h if the blood count is normal and the cultures are negative. The normal I:T ratio on a CBC is less than 0.3:1. Relapse can occur and an infant who has been treated should be carefully examined before discharge, with a repeat CRP and CBC.

REFERENCES

1. Thomsen AC, Morup L, Hansen KB. Antibiotic elimination of group B streptococci in urine in prevention of preterm labour. *Lancet* 1987;i:591–3
2. Allen UD, Navas L, King S. Effectiveness of intrapartum penicillin prophylaxis in preventing early onset group B streptococcal infection: results of a meta-analysis. *Can Med Assoc J* 1993;149:1659–65
3. American Academy of Pediatrics Committee on Infectious Diseases and Committee on Fetus and Newborn. Guidelines for prevention of group B streptococcal infection by chemoprophylaxis. *Pediatrics* 1992;90:775–8
4. Boyer KM, Gotoff SP. Prevention of early onset neonatal group B streptococcal disease with selective intrapartum chemoprophylaxis. *N Engl J Med* 1986;314:1665–9
5. CDC. Prevention of perinatal group B streptococcal disease: a public health perspective. *MMWR Weekly* 1996;45:RR-7
6. Van Oppen C, Feldman R. Antibiotic prophylaxis of neonatal group B streptococcal infection. *Br Med J* 1993;306:411–12
7. Pylipow M, Gaddis M, Kinney JS. Selective intrapartum prophylaxis for group B streptococcus colonization: management and outcome of newborns. *Pediatrics* 1994;93:631–5
8. Society of Obstetricians and Gynaecologists of Canada and Canadian Paediatric Society. National consensus statement on the prevention of early onset group B streptococcal infections in the newborn. *J Soc Obstetr Gynaecol Canada Canadian Paediatr Soc* 1994;16:2271–8
9. Steele RW. Control of neonatal group B streptococcal infection. *J Roy Soc Med* 1993;86:712–15
10. Rouse DJ, Goldenberg RL, Cliver SP, Cutter GR, Mennemeyer ST, Fargason CA. Strategies for the prevention of early onset group B streptococcal sepsis: a decision analysis. *Obstet Gynaecol* 1994;83:483–94
11. Smaill F. Intrapartum antibiotics for GBS colonization. In Neilson JP, ed. *Pregnancy and childbirth module of the Cochrane database of systematic reviews*. Issue 3. Oxford: Update Software, 1997

17

Eclampsia and pre-eclampsia

INTRODUCTION

It should be emphasized that it is likely to be a very stressful time for both the woman who develops pre-eclampsia and her partner. Careful explanation and reassurance by a senior member of the obstetric staff will help to ease much of the anxiety.

SIGNS AND SYMPTOMS ASSOCIATED WITH PRE-ECLAMPSIA

The signs and symptoms of pre-eclampsia are many and include: visual disturbance; flashing lights; headache; epigastric pain; raised blood pressure (BP) ($\geq$ 140 mmHg systolic or $\geq$ 90 mmHg diastolic); hyper-reflexia; clonus (> 2 beats); changes in optic fundi (often very difficult to detect); epigastric or liver edge tenderness; and oedema.

However, it should be noted that headache is a common symptom in pregnancy and conversely that eclamptic fits may occur without any of the above signs or symptoms.

BLOOD PRESSURE RECORDING

BP should be recorded with the cuff at the level of the heart. The diastolic pressure is taken as abolition of heart sounds. The BP should be taken with a large cuff if the arm circumference exceeds 35 cm (often the case in women > 100 kg).

SEVERE PRE-ECLAMPSIA PROTOCOL

Criteria for managing women using this protocol

This protocol is used when the decision has been made to expedite delivery, plus any of the following (A, B or C):

A. Hypertension (> 140/90) with proteinuria (> 0.5 g/l or > 2+) and at least one of the following: significant headache, visual disturbance, epigastric pain; clonus (> 2 beats); or platelet count < 100×10^9, aspartate aminotransferase (AST) > 40 IU/L

B. Severe hypertension (systolic BP > 170 mmHg or diastolic BP > 110 mmHg) with proteinuria (> 2 g/day or > 2+)

C. Eclampsia

If these criteria are met, the patient is managed according to the following protocol irrespective of the mode of delivery or method of analgesia.

Basic organization and observations

The on-call consultant obstetrician, senior specialist registrar and obstetric anaesthetist are informed. Throughout, the woman is nursed in a spacious room on the labour ward. The managing team should commence an intensive care/high-dependency unit observation chart. Blood is taken for measurement of full blood count, urea and electrolytes, liver function tests (LFT), uric acid, platelets, clotting screen, group and save (crossmatching if haemoglobin is low). Serum glucose should be checked if LFT values are abnormal. A blood film should be requested if HELLP (haemolysis, elevated liver enzymes, low platelets) syndrome is suspected. Urine should be collected and sent for urgent microscopy and culture/sensitivities.

Strict fluid balance must be maintained throughout and continued for 2–4 days after delivery. Urine output measurement and urinalysis should be performed hourly. BP measurements should be taken every 15 min using an automated blood pressure recorder and checked manually using a sphigmomanometer and stethoscope every hour. A central venous line may be inserted by the anaesthetist, preferably using a Drum-Cath via the antecubital fossa.

ANTI-HYPERTENSIVE THERAPY

Hydralazine

An intravenous (IV) bolus of 5 mg is given over 5 min. If a reduction in diastolic BP to a mean arterial pressure (MAP) of < 125 mmHg and < 100 mmHg diastolic is not achieved within 20 min, further 5–10 mg increments are given by slow IV bolus until this is achieved. If the MAP remains above 125 mmHg and the pulse rate is > 120/min or 20 mg of hydralazine in total has been given, the labetalol protocol should be followed.

Maintenance treatment with hydralazine is continued using a continuous infusion via a syringe pump (hydralazine 60 mg diluted to 60 ml with 0.9% sodium chloride). The infusion is commenced at a rate of 5 ml/h (5 mg/h) and should be titrated against the maternal blood pressure to achieve a MAP of < 125 mmHg and < 100 mmHg diastolic BP.

If no syringe pumps are available, an Ivac or other volumetric delivery system may be used (hydralazine 80 mg diluted into sodium chloride 1000 ml), but should be replaced with a syringe pump as soon as one becomes available. The infusion is commenced at a rate of 20 drop/min or 60 ml/h (4.8 mg/h) and the dose titrated against the maternal blood pressure to achieve a MAP of < 125 mmHg and < 100 mmHg diastolic BP.

Post-delivery the hydralazine should be reduced after 4 h by 1mg/h. If the BP rises during this reduction nifedipine 5–10 mg sublingually may be used as required to control BP. If sublingual nifedipine is needed, consideration should be given to starting regular oral antihypertensives, such as nifedipine or labetalol. Methyldopa should be avoided post-delivery because of its mood-lowering side-effects.

Labetalol

Labetalol is only to be used in the circumstances above. The consultant on call must be informed if this is required. Labetalol 25 mg IV is given over a least 1 min followed at 10 min intervals by 50, 50 and 75 mg up to a maximum of 200 mg. A maintenance infusion may then be used. Dilute 200 mg in 50 ml saline and start rate at 20 mg/h, doubling every 30 min until a satisfactory response has been achieved or to a maximum of 160 mg/h. Contraindications to labetalol include asthma, heart block and heart failure.

ANTICONVULSANT THERAPY

Magnesium sulphate

An IV bolus of magnesium sulphate 4 g is given over 5 min (diluted in 20 ml 5% dextrose or 0.9% sodium chloride). This is followed by a maintenance infusion via a syringe pump, the solution made up as 20 g magnesium sulphate in 60 ml of 0.9% saline infused at a rate of 3 ml/h (1 g/h). It can be continued at this rate unless the knee jerks are abolished, urine output falls below 50 ml in 2 h or if the respiratory rate falls below 16/min. If urine output falls below 50 ml in 2 h, the obstetric specialist registrar should be contacted. Magnesium administration *must* be stopped if oliguria persists.

Contraindications include cardiac disease and acute renal failure (IV diazepam should be used instead: 10 mg then 2.5 mg/h). The infusion should continue as long as the patient is on the labour ward (i.e. until 24–48 h post-delivery).

Clinical monitoring should involve: tendon reflexes after loading and then hourly (use reflexes at elbow or wrist in patients who have a working epidural); respiratory rate hourly (should be > 16/min); pulse oximetry continuously; level of consciousness hourly

Magnesium levels should be checked or if toxicity is suspected or the infusion is continued for more than 48 h. They need to be checked every 2–4 h if urine output is low (≤ 100 ml/h over 4 h) or if urea is greater than 10 mmol/l or alanine aminotransferase or AST is more than 250 IU/l.

The normal therapeutic level of magnesium in the serum is 2–4 mmol/l. Nausea, a feeling of warmth, weakness, double vision and slurred speech usually occur at a dose of 5 mmol/l, muscle paralysis and respiratory arrest occur at 6–7.5 mmol/l, and cardiac arrest occurs at more than 12 mmol/l.

The maintenance infusion should be terminated and urgent magnesium levels should be sent off and the anaesthetist informed if:

- the patellar reflex is lost

- the respiratory rate is less than 12/min or

- oxygen saturation is persistently less than 95% on air or oxygen

The antidote to magnesium is 1 g of calcium gluconate (10 ml of 10% solution) given IV over 3 min. If cardiac arrest occurs as a result of $MgSO_4$ treatment, calcium gluconate should be given at the same time as cardiopulmonary resuscitation and the crash call is instituted.

MIDWIFERY CARE FOR WOMEN ON PIH PROTOCOL

All women will remain on labour ward for a minimum of 24 h after delivery. This is especially important as 40% of eclamptic fits occur after delivery. Please ensure that when the patient is transferred to the postnatal ward, the ward staff are made aware of the need for strict fluid balance until completion of the fourth postnatal day.

Sometimes, the woman's condition may necessitate her transfer to the intensive therapy unit (ITU). On her transfer back to the labour ward, the midwife should inform the duty anaesthetist and the obstetric team of her return.

ASPECTS OF CARE

Airway management
If there is significant oedema of the airway and/or other airway compromise, oxygen sauration should be continuously monitored, the anaesthetic senior specialist registrar informed and admission to intensive care considered.

ITU charts
ITU charts should be filled in at least hourly. The hourly fluid intake (IV and oral), urine output and fluid balance, BP, central venous pressure, oxygen saturation and blood results should all be recorded, filling in important events (e.g. antihypertensive treatment, epidural insertion and top-ups, time of birth and delivery, and blood loss at delivery).

BP measurement
An automated device is advised for BP measurements. Measurements should be made every 15 min and recorded on the ITU chart and checked every hour with a manual sphigmomanometer and stethoscope. Inform the specialist registrar if there are two consecutive readings with a MAP > 125 mmHg or one MAP reading > 140 mmHg.

Fluid intake
The standard IV fluid regimen is 85 ml/h. This must include the fluid contained in any drug infusions. Once oral fluids are established, the hourly oral intake must be taken into account (i.e. if the woman is drinking 50 ml/h, then IV intake must be reduced to appoximately 35 ml/h).

Urine output
Urine output is measured hourly using an urimeter. The obstetric

specialist registrar should be informed if the output falls below 30 ml/h for more than 2 h.

Central venous pressure

Central venous pressure should be recorded at least every hour. The anaesthetist is responsible for the insertion and subsequent care of the central venous line. If there are any concerns regarding central venous pressure measurement, the anaesthetist should be informed. If the central venous pressure is more than 12 cmH_2O or less than 5 cmH_2O, the obstetric senior house officer and the anaesthetic specialist registrar should be contacted immediately.

Magnesium sulphate

Magnesium sulphate is given by IV infusion. The first signs of toxicity are loss of tendon reflexes and respiratory depression. If oxygen saturation falls below 95%, inform the specialist registrar and the anaesthetist. Please note the clinical monitoring required, which is outlined above.

Cord gases

Every attempt must be made to ensure arterial and venous cord samples are taken, and complete results should be recorded in the delivery notes.

ECLAMPSIA

The management of eclampsia should follow a similar pattern to that of severe pre-eclampsia. The eclamptic fit should always be controlled by immediate IV drug therapy, while the woman is placed on her side, in a head down position and given oxygen. IV magnesium sulphate 4 g should be given over 5 min, followed by an infusion of 1 g/h for 24 h. If the convulsions recur, a further bolus of IV magnesium sulphate 4 g should be given. In the event of further convulsions, IV diazepam (at least 10 mg) should be given. In all cases the paediatrician must be informed of all medication the mother has received, as it may affect the neonate's condition.

In the presence of severe pre-eclampsia or following an eclamptic fit, the primary objective is assessment and stabilization of the woman's condition before proceeding to delivery, since anaesthesia and surgery immediately after a fit can compromise the maternal condition. Results of clotting studies, LFTs, platelet count and clotting should be made available as soon as possible.

MODE OF DELIVERY

A long labour is contraindicated in women with pre-eclampsia, and lower segment Caesarean section should be performed sooner rather than later. If labour progresses quickly, a spontaneous vaginal delivery – aided if necessary by an episiotomy – may be achieved. Prolonged pushing may generate further rises in BP. Instrumental delivery is indicated if the second stage does not proceed quickly.

ANALGESIA IN LABOUR

Epidural analgesia can be extremely beneficial in the management of labour complicated by pre-eclampsia. It lowers the BP in pre-eclamptic women, although it may not abolish BP peaks. The rise in BP associated with painful uterine contractions is attenuated, and adequate analgesia/anaesthesia is easily provided for the likely forceps or Caesarean delivery. However, this technique is contraindicated in the presence of significant abnormalities of platelet count or clotting screen. Care must be taken to anticipate and prevent an excessive fall in BP, usually by means of judicious crystalloid/colloid pre-loading.

THE THIRD STAGE

IV syntocinon 10 units should be given following delivery. Syntometrine or ergometrine must not be given, as their administration will raise BP and may cause stroke.

The woman should be kept under close observation for at least 24 h after delivery. Antihypertensive treatment should be reduced progressively, but it must be remembered that the condition may initially worsen in the immediate postpartum period. Magnesium sulphate therapy should be continued until the reflexes are normal, the BP has settled, and the proteinuria has cleared. Typically, this will occur within 24 h, but in some circumstances treatment may need to be continued.

Post-delivery the hydralazine dose should be reduced after 4 h by 1 mg/h. If the BP rises during this period, nifedipine 5–10 mg sublingually may be used as required to control it. If sublingual nifedipine is needed, consideration should be given to starting regular oral antihypertensives, such as labetalol or nifedipine.

EXCEPTIONAL CIRCUMSTANCES

As a general rule, women requiring antihypertensive therapy for proteinuric hypertension should also have anticonvulsant therapy. However, when there is significant hypertension in the absence of hyperflexia, as occurs in some cases of essential hypertension, then antihypertensive therapy may be given alone.

BIBLIOGRAPHY

Clements RV. *Safe Practice in Obstetrics and Gynaecology.* Edinburgh: Churchill Livingstone, 1994:492

Edmonds DK, ed. *Dewhurst's Textbook of Obstetrics and Gynaecology for Postgraduates,* Sixth edition. Oxford: Blackwell Science, 1999:622

James DK, *et al. High Risk Pregnancy.* London: WB Saunders, 1994:1318

18

Management of maternal diabetes in labour

INTRODUCTION

The management plan outlined in this chapter applies equally to women with established diabetes as well as to those with gestational diabetes, except where specifically stated below. During pregnancy, diabetic women are generally cared for in a combined obstetric/diabetic clinic.

ON ADMISSION TO THE LABOUR WARD

The obstetric and diabetes specialist registrars should be informed of the labouring diabetic woman's admission to the labour ward. An intravenous (IV) insulin and glucose infusion should be started: dextrose 5% 1000 ml 12-hourly with 40 mmol potassium in each litre and 50 units human Actrapid made up in 50 ml saline (1 unit/ml). Blood glucose levels should ideally be kept between 4 and 7 mmol/l. If a Caesarean section is planned, the woman should fast from midnight and commence the IV regimen 6 h later.

CALCULATION OF THE INSULIN DOSE

If glucose control prior to labour has been kept in the range 7.1–10 the total daily insulin dose is calculated using the following formula:

Calculated Daily dose = Long + Short acting insulin

This figure is divided by 24 to give hourly insulin requirement.

Blood glucose (BG) level should be tested hourly, adjusting the hourly rate according to the following scale:

BG < 4 = 25% calculated hourly requirement

BG 4–7 = 50% calculated hourly requirement

BG 7.1–10 = calculated hourly requirement

BG 10.1–15 = 150% calculated hourly requirement

BG 15.1–28 = 200% calculated hourly requirement

BG > 28 = 400% calculated hourly requirement

Women who have diet-controlled diabetes should have 1–2 hourly blood glucose monitoring and have an insulin infusion started if the blood glucose rises above 11 mmol/l.

INSULIN REQUIREMENT POST-DELIVERY

Women with established diabetes should have their insulin dose reduced by 50% at delivery of placenta. They should be converted to a subcutaneous regimen when eating and drinking normally. Insulin should be stopped post-delivery in those women in whom the diagnosis of gestational diabetes is clear.

FOLLOW-UP APPOINTMENTS

Before discharge

It is recommended that before discharge, women with established diabetes should have an appointment made for an outpatient clinic 6 weeks post-discharge (or sooner if necessary) after delivery, while women with gestational diabetes should have an OGGT 6 weeks after delivery.

CARE OF THE BABY

The baby will be seen and examined by the paediatrician at birth and, as with all other deliveries, a sample of venous and arterial cord blood will be obtained following delivery and the following tests performed: packed cell volume, haematocrit, glucose levels and blood gases.

Chapter 8 of this book covers the management of the infant at high risk of hypoglycaemia. Symptoms of hypoglycaemia should be carefully looked for in the first few days postpartum, especially lethargy, poor feeding, apnoea, rolling eye movements and fits. The paediatrician should be informed promptly if hypoglycaemia is suspected.

RECORDS

A copy of the computer delivery printout should be placed in the diabetic notes before discharge.

BIBLIOGRAPHY

Clements RV. Safe Practice in Obstetrics and Gynaecology. Edinburgh: Churchill Livingstone, 1994:492

De Swiet M, ed. *Medical Disorders in Obstetric Practice*, 4th edn. Oxford: Blackwell Science, 1995:683

Edmonds DK, ed. *Dewhurst's Textbook of Obstetrics and Gynaecology for Postgraduates*, Sixth edition. Oxford: Blackwell Science, 1999:622

James DK, *et al. High Risk Pregnancy*. London: WB Saunders, 1994:1318

Maresh M. Diabetes in pregnancy. *Contemp Clin Gynecol Obstet* 2001;1:243–54

19

Infection control precautions with particular reference to women with blood-borne pathogens (hepatitis B or HIV)

Because it is not always possible to know when a woman is carrying blood-borne pathogens, staff must practise good infection control techniques at all times. When a known HIV- or hepatitis B-positive woman is in labour, it is important that the staff caring for the woman and her partner are sensitive to the couple's situation whilst implementing the precautions necessary to minimize the risk of infection to staff. Time should be taken to explain to the woman and her partner why these precautions are necessary and they should be carried out as discretely as possible.

All staff working on the labour ward should familiarize themselves with the infection control policy and ensure that they maintain the standards defined. In addition to these standards, the following additional precautions must be undertaken when a woman is known to be highly infectious:

- Invasive procedures that impose risk of infection to the fetus, such as fetal blood sampling and the use of scalp electrodes should not be used unless specifically requested by the consultant in charge

- Masks and eye protection should be worn by all involved in the delivery and operative procedures

- Latex gloves should be worn for receiving the baby and throughout the initial examination. Providing the baby is well and warm, he/she should be bathed as soon as possible after delivery to remove any blood or secretions. Until this is done the person handling the baby should wear gloves and a plastic apron

- Once the mother and baby have been washed, protective clothing may be discarded. However, for any procedures involving material or apparatus stained with blood or body fluids, gloves and plastic aprons should be worn

- All blood-stained linen including any of the baby's should be sent to the laundry in a green alginate stitched bag and an outer green or clear plastic bag

- All disposable items should be placed in yellow plastic bags for incineration

When a Caesarean section is required in a highly infectious patient, the following should also be undertaken:

- To reduce the need for cleaning up large amounts of blood, it is recommended that the swab rack and trough are draped with a polythene sheet that can be rolled up together with all the swabs after the count and discarded

- Double latex gloves should be worn by the operator

- A special sticky discard pad should be used for needles and blades and should be placed in the sharps bin after the count. Each member of the team is responsible for rinsing body fluids off their own boots and goggles in the sluice at the end of the case

- Protective clothing must be worn when washing blood and secretions off instruments and equipment

MANAGEMENT OF WOMEN IN LABOUR WHO ARE HIV-POSITIVE WHO HAVE EITHER NOT ATTENDED BEFORE OR ATTENDED SPORADICALLY

Details should be obtained of previous test results and any current treatment for HIV. If the woman is taking antiretroviral medication, perhaps from another hospital, it should be continued. If in doubt, the HIV specialist team should be consulted.

Baseline blood tests

Take blood for full blood count, biochemical screen, confirmatory HIV test (if the patient has not attended the hospital before), viral load and CD4 count (please add additional antenatal bloods).

Antiretroviral drugs

Give intravenous zidovudine to mother as below:

Consider single dose nevirapine (200 mg) to mother during labour. This can result in antiretroviral resistance unless additional drugs are given, and so should not be used unless the mother is likely to take additional drugs in the next week. If so, give the mother zidovudine 250 mg twice-daily, didanosine 400 mg at night (at least 2 h after food) for 7 days.

Delivery

The use of Caesarean section should be discussed with the mother as the optimal mode of delivery. Even in the presence of prolonged ruptured membranes lower segment Caesarean section will still reduce the risk of vertical transmission. If the mother refuses a Caesarean section then avoid any obstetric interventions. Do not perform an artificial rupture of the membranes. If the cardiotocogram becomes abnormal discuss again the use of Caesarean section. Under no circumstances should a fetal scalp electrode be applied or a fetal blood sample be performed. If any such women are admitted to the labour ward, their management should be discussed with the consultant.

Drugs for the baby

Zidovudine is given routinely as per the routine protocol. If the mother has been given a single dose of nevirapine, the baby should then also be given a single dose (see below).

Follow-up

Following delivery, the woman must be seen by a member of the specialist HIV team who will make suitable follow-up arrangements. It should be ensured that the woman has a postnatal appointment to see the relevant obstetric consultant.

MANAGEMENT OF INFANTS BORN TO HIV-POSITIVE MOTHERS

Delivery and postnatal examination

When attending the delivery of an infant born to an HIV-positive mother, universal infection control procedures should be observed with the handling of all body fluid from the mother and the infant. The mother will usually have been counselled not to breast feed the infant, as it is known that breast feeding increases the risk of transmission of HIV from mother to child by 100%. In all cases bottle feeding will be recommended. It is most unusual for mothers to elect to breast feed the infant when they have been given this information.

The baby should have the normal neonatal examination performed in the usual way. The examiner should wear gloves when testing the sucking reflex. It is not necessary to wear gloves for the rest of the examination. The neonatal specialist registrar and consultant should be notified that an infant has been born to an HIV-positive mother, because the baby's antiretroviral treatment should start without delay.

KING'S COLLEGE PROTOCOL FOR THE ADMINISTRATION OF ANTI-RETROVIRAL MEDICATION TO HIV-POSITIVE WOMEN DURING CHILDBIRTH AND THEIR INFANTS

Please note that this protocol is intended as a guide only. Decisions regarding choice of therapy for individual patients should rest with the consultant responsible for those patients' care.

Contents of maternity zidovudine pack

Pre-prepared packs contain:

- 5 × zidovudine vials (200 mg/20 ml)

- 1 × 500 ml 5% dextrose solution

- 1 × 100 ml 5% dextrose solution

- 1 × 200 ml zidovudine syrup 10 mg/ml and oral syringe

There is a label on the outside of the pack upon which the midwife or pharmacist should write the patient's name and hospital number before the medicine is administered. Once allocated to a patient the pack should stay with that patient during all stages of their care within the hospital.

Maternal zidovudine administration

The intravenous zidovudine is already in solution. Each vial contains 200 mg in 20 ml. This must be diluted with 5% dextrose prior to administration.

A loading dose of 2 mg/kg should be given. For example, a patient weighing 70 kg requires a dose of 140 mg. Each vial contains 200 mg of zidovudine in 20 ml, therefore a volume of 14 ml is needed. Add the required volume to a 100 ml bag of 5% dextrose and infuse over 60 min.

Maintenance

The maintenance infusion can be prepared at the same time as the loading dose infusion. This infusion should be given at a rate of 1 mg/kg/h and is normally given over 12 h or until delivery.

For example, a 70 kg patient would require 70 mg/h or 840 mg over 12 h. For this patient a volume of 84 ml (840 mg) should be added to 500 ml of 5% dextrose and the infusion should be given for 12 h or until delivery.

Part-used or unused packs must be returned to pharmacy.

Neonatal zidovudine

The antiretroviral pack contains a 200 ml bottle of zidovudine syrup 10 mg/ml. This is intended for the newborn infant and so must be sent to the ward with the mother following delivery. The ward pharmacist will complete the label by writing the correct dose, in ml, to be administered to the infant. Other information on the bottle should not be obscured or changed in any way during the infant's admission.

Neonatal zidovudine administration

Zidovudine syrup should be given to the infant at a dose of 2 mg/kg body weight, orally, four times a day. The first dose should be given within 1 h of birth and treatment should be continued for 6 weeks. Zidovudine may be administered by the mother or senior midwife and double-checked by a second midwife. The medicine should be stored in a medicine cupboard at all other times and must only be used for the infant to which it has been allocated. In certain cases where a mother is administering the medicine to her child it may be allowable to keep the medicine in a locked cupboard in the mother's room. This must be agreed with the ward pharmacist.

For infants who are unable to take oral medication, the zidovudine can be given intravenously. In this case the dose is 1.5 mg/kg body weight four times daily.

Dose adjustments for infants born before 34 weeks
A dose adjustment is required for infants born very prematurely. The zidovudine doses for these infants should be calculated as follows: 1.5 mg/kg body weight every 12 h from birth until 2 weeks of age. After 2 weeks of age increase dose to 2 mg/kg body weight every 8 h. Treatment should be continued for 6 weeks post delivery.

Supply of medication upon discharge
When the mother and baby are due to go home a prescription should be written for zidovudine 2 mg/kg four times daily continuing for 6 weeks after birth. The zidovudine syrup on the ward may be used for the home use providing that a pharmacist checks it and that the dose in ml is written on the label. If the ward pharmacist has not checked the medicine then it must be brought to dispensary with the prescription so that it can be checked.

Nevirapine
On the advice of a consultant, a single dose of nevirapine is sometimes given to the infant 48–72 h post delivery. The dose required is 2 mg/kg body weight. The ward pharmacist will make up the medicine in an oral syringe on an individual basis for each infant. The syringe will contain the exact dose required and will be labelled appropriately.

BIBLIOGRAPHY

Clements RV. *Safe Practice in Obstetrics and Gynaecology*. Edinburgh: Churchill Livingstone, 1994:492

Ravizza M, Mangiarotti L, Della Grazia S, Foina S, Pardi G. HIV in pregnancy. *Contemp Clin Gynecol Obstet* 2001;1:49–58

20

Management of shoulder dystocia

ANTICIPATION

Shoulder dystocia should be suspected in the presence of a variety of risk factors including: recognized macrosomia of present pregnancy (> 4 kg); previous shoulder dystocia (recurrence risk is approximately 15%) or large baby (> 4 kg); diabetes mellitus (DM); or maternal obesity.

When risk factors such as fetal macrosomia, DM or previous shoulder dystocia have been identified, the specialist registrar on call should be on the labour ward and available during the second stage of labour. This should be recorded clearly in the patient's notes.

The normal procedure of aspirating mucus from the baby's mouth and correcting a nuchal cord should be undertaken at delivery.

Shoulder dystocia is significant if the head-to-body delivery time is more than 5 min or if any of the procedures below are needed.

DRILL

Help should be summoned in the form of the most experienced obstetric doctor and an anaesthetist. The woman should be placed in

McRoberts' position with sharp hyperreflexion of the thighs onto the abdomen held by two assistants, or in the all-fours position. A mediolateral episiotomy must be done, or liberally extended if it has already been done. Pressure is exerted suprapubically to dislodge the anterior shoulder. This should be applied with the palm of the hand just to the side of the midline to the side to which the baby is facing. The pressure should be posterior and lateral to achieve a rotation pressure. At the same time the head and neck should be pushed posteriorly from below. A common error is to apply strong downward and rotation pressure at this point. It is important that the pressure should be smooth and continuous avoiding the application of sudden jerks. This effort should be made for 5–10 s, but if it fails it is wise to desist and attempt other manoeuvres. The woman should be discouraged from pushing indiscriminately during this time as this may only increase impaction of the shoulders. Fundal pressure is contraindicated.

Most situations will be resolved by the above procedure. For those that are not resolved, the collaboration of an anaesthetist becomes important, particularly if there is no pre-existing epidural block. Wood's manouvre or the manoeuvre to deliver the posterior shoulder may be used next, in the order preferred by the most senior obstetrician present.

Wood's manoeuvre
When anaesthesia is adequate, manipulation should be undertaken to rotate the shoulders using Wood's manoeuvre. An attempt should be made to rotate the shoulders through 180° using two fingers from each hand on the baby's shoulders. The posterior shoulder is thereby rotated anteriorly and in front of the symphysis pubis. Care must be taken to manipulate the shoulder and not the head. Both the shoulders should move forwards towards the chest thereby reducing the bisacrominal diameter.

Delivery of the posterior shoulder
An attempt should be made to deliver the posterior shoulder. Anaesthesia is necessary to facilitate passage of the hand into the posterior part of the birth canal. If the fetal back is on the right then the operator's right hand is used and vice versa. The operator reaches for the posterior shoulder. The upper arm is then followed to the elbow. A finger is passed into the antecubital fossa to encourage flexion of the elbow joint. As the operator's hand is passed further down the fetal forearm, the wrist or hand can be felt. An attempt can then be made to sweep the forearm over the fetal chest and deliver the posterior arm.

The bisacromial diameter is therefore then reduced and the delivery of the rest of the baby follows.

These manouvres may cause clavicular or humerus fractures, but these usually heal well and are preferable to nerve root avulsions resulting from traction on the fetal head.

If these methods fail, the senior specialist registrar or consultant should attempt the Zavanelli manoeuvre.

Zavanelli manoeuvre

The Zavanelli manoeuvre involves repositioning of the head under anaesthesia and delivery by Caesarean section (CS). The procedure is as follows: the patient is prepared for CS delivery; a bolus dose of tocolytic (terbutaline 0.25 mg) is given subcutaneously; a scalp electrode is then applied, checking fetal heart; and the head is pushed back into the vagina in an occiput anterior position. The head must be re-flexed and kept in the position of flexion and the vertex pushed upwards. This position must be maintained until delivery by CS.

POST-DELIVERY

The vagina and cervix should be carefully examined to assess and repair any damage. Cord gases (both an aterial and venous sample) should also be taken.

BIBLIOGRAPHY

Clements RV. *Safe Practice in Obstetrics and Gynaecology.* Edinburgh: Churchill Livingstone, 1994:492

Edmonds DK, ed. *Dewhurst's Textbook of Obstetrics and Gynaecology for Postgraduates,* Sixth edition. Oxford: Blackwell Science, 1999:622

James DK, *et al. High Risk Pregnancy.* London: WB Saunders, 1994:1318

21

Breech delivery

The consultant on call for the labour ward should be made aware of any labouring woman with a breech presentation and of the intended maternal position for vaginal delivery.

INTENDED DELIVERY POSITION

The decision to adopt a delivery position other than lithotomy should have been discussed in the antenatal clinic with the relevant consultant. If this has not occurred, the consultant on call should be made aware. Until the results of more studies of standing breech delivery are available, it is not recommended. Anecdotal reports suggest a high risk of fetal morbidity and mortality.

FIRST STAGE OF LABOUR

The labour and analgesia provisions for women with breech presentation are identical to women with vertex presentation. If the breech is engaged and the admission cardiotocograph (CTG) is satisfactory, the baby's condition may be monitored intermittently according to the protocol for normal labour. The National Institute for Clinical Excellence/ Royal College of Obstetricians and Gynaecologists recommendations[1] are that continuous electronic fetal monitoring should be used. This should always be discussed with the woman prior to its use (see page 23).

A vaginal examination is always performed immediately after rupture of membranes for the following reasons:

- to exclude cord prolapse

- to ascertain whether the breech is complete or incomplete

- to determine dilatation of the cervix

- to assess the station of the breech and

- to assess pelvic size

If there are any fetal heart decelerations, the fetal heart rate should be monitored continuously using an electronic fetal monitor. If the quality of the CTG is poor from the external transducer, it may be necessary to continue monitoring via an electrode attached to the fetal buttock, which should be attached by a senior specialist registrar. If fetal compromise is suspected, the senior obstetric specialist registrar should be informed.

SECOND STAGE OF LABOUR

If continuous electronic fetal monitoring is not in progress during the second stage of labour, the midwife should listen to the baby's heart rate using an ultrasound transducer after every contraction once pushing starts. All values should be recorded. If the auscultated fetal heart rate gives cause for concern then a continuous record must be obtained using an electronic fetal monitor.

BIRTH OF THE BABY

It is essential that the consultant on call is aware of the delivery and that a consultant or senior specialist registrar is present at delivery, which should be conducted in a large delivery room near the theatres or in theatre. An appropriately experienced paediatrician should also be present and resuscitation equipment made ready. Cord gases (both arterial and venous) should be taken.

THE NEWLY DIAGNOSED ('UNDIAGNOSED') BREECH

The senior specialist registrar should be informed of any woman admitted with a newly diagnosed breech presentation and should then review and examine the woman and discuss futher mangement in detail. The case should be discussed with the consultant on call.

Examination

An estimation of fetal weight should be made clinically or using ultrasound, while clinical pelvimetry may be performed to assess the true conjugate, sacral curve, intertuberous distance and subpubic arch.

REFERENCE

1. *The Use of Electronic Fetal Monitoring: the Use and Interpretation of Cardiotocography in Intrapartum Fetal Surveillance* (Guideline no. 8). London: RCOG Press, 2001

BIBLIOGRAPHY

Clements RV. *Safe Practice in Obstetrics and Gynaecology.* Edinburgh: Churchill Livingstone, 1994:492

Edmonds DK, ed. *Dewhurst's Textbook of Obstetrics and Gynaecology for Postgraduates*, Sixth edition. Oxford: Blackwell Science, 1999:622

James DK, *et al.* High Risk Pregnancy. London: WB Saunders, 1994:1318

22

Twin delivery

The aim is to allow the woman with term twins to deliver them safely with minimum intervention but with experienced personnel present. On the woman's admission, the senior house officer (SHO) and specialist registrar should be informed. If labour is confirmed, the senior specialist registrar should be informed and should review the woman, informing the consultant on call. For the purposes of training junior staff at King's College Hospital, the consultant on call should be present at all twin deliveries occurring between 09:00 and 17:00. A scan should be performed to determine lie, position and fetal heart rates. When the second stage commences, the midwife should inform the duty SHO who will, in turn, inform the specialist registrars, anaesthetist and paediatrician.

Continuous monitoring should be strongly recommended throughout labour in preterm twins and in a complicated twin pregnancy at whatever gestation. It should continue throughout the second stage in all twins at whatever gestation. If there is any doubt whether both fetal hearts are being recorded or the quality of the cardiotocogram of either twin is poor, then a scalp electrode should be used for one twin and an external monitor for the other.

Twin delivery should be conducted in a large delivery room near to theatres. The following personnel should be present: obstetric senior specialist registrar and SHO; suitably experienced paediatricians; anaesthetist (and anaesthetic nurse/ODA); and sufficient midwifery staff.

For second stage management the following should be prepared:

- Intravenous cannula *in situ* (blood taken for full blood count and group and save serum)

- Infusion of 1000 ml saline plus syntocinon 8 IU for augmentation of second stage (this should be prepared but not connected)

- Infusion for syringe pump containing syntocinon 20 IU in 50 ml or 100 ml saline or 1000 ml saline plus syntocinon 40 IU for postpartum (this should be prepared, clearly labelled, but not connected)

- Ultrasound (US) monitor

- Ventouse and forceps packs

- Two resuscitaires and extra cord clamps

If twin 1 is cephalic with normal progress and normal fetal position, the midwife should deliver this twin in the usual manner. However, if twin 1 is a breech presentation, delivery will be conducted with the woman in lithotomy by medical personnel or midwifery staff under medical supervision. After delivery of twin 1, the cord is clamped with a single cord clamp and the baby handed to a paediatrician.

It is necessary for the medical team to ensure the following:

- Check presentation of the second twin by abdominal palpation and with ultrasound. Specialist registrar to maintain longitudinal lie of baby until contractions recommence. If lie is transverse, external version to a cephalic presentation is preferable

- Ensure fetal heart rate is satisfactory by carefully repositioning the monitor with the aid of US, if necessary

If contractions have not recommenced after 5 min, syntocinon infusion (syntocinon 8 U in 1000 ml Hartman's solution) should be commenced at 30 ml/h and increased by 30 ml/h at 5 min intervals to a maximum of 180 ml/h or until contractions are satisfactory. The mother should be encouraged to commence active pushing when contractions are satisfactory.

The delivery of the second twin should not be rushed if all is normal. The membranes of the second amniotic sac should not be ruptured until the presenting part is well down the pelvis. The interval between delivery of twins 1 and 2 is usually less than 30 min but may be up to 1 h if the fetal and maternal condition is satisfactory. The planned interval between vaginal deliveries should not be more than 1 h.

If the second twin is cephalic, delivery should be by the midwife in the usual way. If the second twin is in a breech presentation, delivery should be conducted with the woman in the lithotomy position by medical personnel or midwifery staff under medical supervision.

Artificial rupture of the second sac of the membranes should be performed only if the presenting part is in the pelvis and advancing and contractions are satisfactory. If after 30 min pushing, delivery is not imminent then instrumental delivery should be considered. After delivery of the second twin the cord should be marked with two cord clamps.

Cord gases (both aterial and venous samples) should be taken from both cords. Intramuscular syntocinin 10 IU should be given after delivery of the second twin and the postpartum syntocinon infusion (via a syringe pump or giving set) commenced at 10 IU/h for 1 h following delivery.

PRETERM DELIVERY OF TWINS

The senior specialist registrar and consultant on call for labour ward must be involved with all decision making regarding the delivery of preterm twins.

BIBLIOGRAPHY

Clements RV. *Safe Practice in Obstetrics and Gynaecology*. Edinburgh: Churchill Livingstone, 1994:492

Edmonds DK, ed. *Dewhurst's Textbook of Obstetrics and Gynaecology for Postgraduates*, Sixth edition. Oxford: Blackwell Science, 1999:622

James DK, *et al. High Risk Pregnancy*. London: WB Saunders, 1994:1318

23

Prolapse of the umbilical cord

INTRODUCTION

Immediate vaginal or speculum examination should be carried out following membrane rupture in the following pregnancy risk groups:

- cardiotocographic abnormality
- unengaged presenting part
- malpresentation (including breech)
- prematurity
- multiple pregnancy and
- polyhydramnios

Be aware that pronounced slowing of the fetal heart may not necessarily accompany cord prolapse.

MANAGEMENT OF CASES OF PROLAPSE OF THE UMBILICAL CORD

Immediate delivery of the baby is required in all cases of umbilical cord prolapse. The obstetric specialist registrar, an anaesthetist and paediatrician should all be summoned immediately, while positioning the woman in the knee-chest or exaggerated Sims position. The presenting part should be pushed upwards to relieve pressure on the cord (with a sterile gloved hand in the vagina); this is continued until delivery of the baby commences. The cord should then be replaced in the vagina if needed, but not through the cervix. Explanation and reassurance should be given to the woman (and her partner). Blood should be taken for urgent group and save serum or cross-matching if Caesarean section (CS) is to be performed.

If the cervix is fully dilated and the head is low, ventouse or forceps delivery may be performed. If the cervix is not fully dilated, CS should be undertaken unless the fetus is dead or very premature, depending on circumstances. Failure to detect pulsation in the cord usually indicates fetal death but ultrasound confirmation must be obtained.

BIBLIOGRAPHY

Clements RV. *Safe Practice in Obstetrics and Gynaecology*. Edinburgh: Churchill Livingstone, 1994:492

Edmonds DK, ed. *Dewhurst's Textbook of Obstetrics and Gynaecology for Postgraduates*, Sixth edition. Oxford: Blackwell Science, 1999:622

24

Uterine rupture

The following signs should be of concern in women who are at risk of uterine rupture:

- cardiotocographic abnormality

- haematuria

- antepartum haemorrhage, however small

- cessation of contractions and

- Bandle's retraction ring

All staff should be aware that: uterine rupture can present as collapse and haemorrhage or it may be 'silent' with no obvious symptoms, and that it may present postpartum.

When a case of uterine rupture presents, labour ward staff should always seek assistance from the senior sister on the labour ward, the senior anaesthetist and/or the senior obstetric specialist registrar. The senior specialist registrar should inform the consultant on call.

The baby should be continuously monitored – if possible a scalp electrode should be placed on the baby's head/bottom. The theatre is prepared and the team should be ready to commence Caesarean section to deliver the baby as soon as possible.

Two large bore (grey) intravenous lines should be inserted, taking bloods for group, cross-match 4 units and clotting studies.

It should be remembered that it may become necessary to follow the procedure for massive haemorrhage (see Chapter 25). Laparotomy/hysterectomy may be necessary, so theatre staff should be prepared for swift operation. Throughout the management of this very rare and serious obstetric emergency, the woman and her family/friends should be informed of what is happening and why.

BIBLIOGRAPHY

Clements RV. *Safe Practice in Obstetrics and Gynaecology*. Edinburgh: Churchill Livingstone, 1994:492

De Swiet M, ed. Medical Disorders in Obstetric Practise, 4th edn. Oxford: Blackwell Science, 1995:683

Edmonds DK, ed. *Dewhurst's Textbook of Obstetrics and Gynaecology for Postgraduates*, Sixth edition. Oxford: Blackwell Science, 1999:622

James DK, *et al. High Risk Pregnancy*. London: WB Saunders, 1994:1318

25

Management of postpartum haemorrhage

DEGREE OF LOSS

It should be noted that blood loss is usually underestimated. All efforts should be made to quantify blood loss objectively, e.g. by weighing swabs.

TABLE 25-1. DEFINITIONS OF POSTPARTUM HAEMORRHAGE

Massive	Loss is > 2 l and is ongoing
Major	Loss is 1–2 l
Moderate	Loss is 0.5–1 l and has ceased

Medical staff must be called and an intravenous cannula inserted if blood loss reaches 1 l and is ongoing. It must always be assumed that blood loss will continue unless it can be shown that it has clearly stopped.

Regardless of blood loss, changes in blood pressure or pulse should prompt referral to hospital or medical attention. If transferred to hospital, all women should have an IV line *in situ*.

CAUSES

The most common cause of postpartum haemorrhage (PPH) is an atonic uterus, but the following must also be considered: retained placenta; a tear of the vaginal wall or cervix; a vulval or paravaginal haematoma; a uterine scar rupture; diffuse intravascular coagulation; and amniotic fluid embolus. Moreover, staff should be aware of concealed bleeding, which may be intrauterine, intraperitoneal, broad ligament and/or paravaginal in origin.

RESUSCITATION

If PPH is major, the cause of the haemorrhage has to be treated and the patient made stable. The sequence of events is as follows:

- Call senior house officer (SHO)
- Insert 16G Venflon
- Send blood for full blood count investigation
- Crossmatch 2 units of whole blood
- Send blood for clotting studies
- Give oxygen by face mask
- Ensure that the womans bladder is empty
- Keep the woman on the labour ward for at least the next 2 h for observation and
- Repeat haemoglobin values the next day

If PPH is massive, the SHO, specialist registrar and anaesthetist should be called (see Chapter 26).

TREATMENT OF ATONIC UTERUS

Staff should perform the following investigations in women who have been shown to have an atonic uterus: check that the placenta is complete and ensure that the woman's bladder is empty. Intravenous (IV) syntocinon 10 IU should be administered and staff should 'rub up' a contraction. If there is no response to this measure, the following sequence should be undertaken (each should be attempted in order if there has been no response to the previous measure):

- Repeat IV syntocinon 10 IU

- IV syntocinon 30 IU in 30 ml N saline at 10 ml/h via a syringe pump or IV syntocinon 50 IU in 500 ml N saline at 100 ml/h via giving set

- Intramyometrial or deep intramuscular prostaglandin F_2/carboprost (Haemabate®) 0.25 mg = 1 ampoule, repeated at intervals of 15 min or more according to response, up to a maximum of 8 ampoules and/or

- Misoprostol 800 µg (four tablets) rectally

If an atonic uterus is not found to be the cause of the PPH, the woman should be managed according to the advice of the senior specialist registrar and/or consultant.

26

Guidelines for the management of massive obstetric haemorrhage

Massive obstetric haemorrhage is defined as sudden, continuing blood loss of 2000 ml or more. All the necessary personnel should be rapidly summoned. These include the senior specialist registrar in obstetrics, the anaesthetic senior specialist registrar and midwives. The specialist registrar in haematology and blood transfusion service should be informed as soon as possible. The anaesthetist and a more senior specialist registrar should assist with the resuscitation and should always be present. The obstetric consultant on call and a senior anaesthetist should be kept fully informed and should be present on the labour ward if haemorrhage is ongoing and exceeds 2500 ml.

Two peripheral infusion lines should be inserted (with at least 16-gauge cannula) into the forearm. Infusion with a compression cuff on the bag is useful. If the patient requires a general anaesthetic, the anaesthetist involved may insert a central venous line.

The blood bank should be informed immediately, giving the patient's name, ward, date of birth and hospital number. Send a blood group/cross-match sample urgently to the blood bank, labelling it appropriately (e.g. "massive bleeding"). A porter should be called to the labour ward. The following investigations should be performed using 20 ml of the woman's blood:

- Cross-match 6 units of blood

- Coagulation studies

- Full blood count

- Urea and electrolytes

A foley catheter should be inserted, with a urimeter recording output hourly. Once the mother is stabilized, a decision should be made about delivery, in consultation with the consultant on-call. If the baby has died following a massive placental abruption, a vaginal examination should be performed, the membranes ruptured and a syntocinon infusion commenced. If the baby is still alive, the mother should be transferred to the operating theatre for immediate delivery. If the haemorrhage occurs after delivery the mother should be transferred to the operating theatre for an examination under anaesthetic.

Whole blood is the treatment of choice but, if necessary, plasma reduced blood may be used in the first instance. Human albumin is preferable, but Haemaccel may be obtained more quickly. Dextran should not be used.

Patients should be transfused with blood of their own group as soon as possible but group O negative should be used if necessary. A supply of O negative blood should be kept on the labour ward for this purpose. If there are any difficulties in obtaining cross-matched blood as top priority from the transfusion service, the haematology consultant on call must be informed immediately.

Infusion with a compression cuff on the bag is useful, and a blood warmer should be used. Following delivery, if the uterus does not respond to conventional treatment, intramyometrial prostaglandins may be used.

BLOOD BANK AND BLOOD PRODUCTS

The blood bank will issue a set combination of blood products, an example of which is shown in Table 26-1.

The blood bank should be notified when the need for massive blood transfusion has ceased or if 'flying squad' blood was used. Unused blood products should always be returned.

If red-cell antibodies are present in the patient's serum, the blood bank technician will alert the physician in charge of the patient and the haematologist, and discuss how to proceed.

TABLE 26-1. PROVISION OF BLOOD PRODUCTS IN MASSIVE BLOOD LOSS

Stage I : 6 units of red cells (RC)

Stage II: 6 units of RC; FFP 15 ml/kg

Stage III: 6 units of RC; one dose of platelets if platelet count < 80 000; FFP 15 ml/kg if prothrombin time or activated partial thromboplastin time ratio is greater than 1.5; Cryoprecipitate 20 units if fibrinogen is less than 1.0 g/l.

OBSERVATIONS

It is essential that an intensive care unit (ICU) chart is maintained throughout the management of patients with massive obstetric haemorrhage, and consideration should be given to transferring the patient to the ICU.

Massive obstetric haemorrhage is one of the most dangerous situations encountered in obstetric practice. It is frightening not only for the staff and the patient (who may remain conscious throughout), but also for the partner. It is essential that one member of staff stays by the woman's side in an attempt to reduce her stress levels. The partner should also be kept fully informed of events.

BIBLIOGRAPHY

Clements RV. *Safe Practice in Obstetrics and Gynaecology.* Edinburgh: Churchill Livingstone, 1994:492

De Swiet M, ed. *Medical Disorders in Obstetric Practise,* 4th edn. Oxford: Blackwell Science, 1995:683

Edmonds DK, ed. *Dewhurst's Textbook of Obstetrics and Gynaecology for Postgraduates,* Sixth edition. Oxford: Blackwell Science, 1999:622

James DK, *et al. High Risk Pregnancy.* London: WB Saunders, 1994:1318

27

Rescue cerclage

INTRODUCTION

Rescue cerclage is performed between 18 and 26 weeks' gestation. The technique in this high-risk situation is difficult and should not be attempted by doctors unfamiliar with the method. The decision should be discussed with the consultant on call.

The woman and her partner must be fully informed regarding the planned procedure and the risk of failure (rupture of membranes, chorioamnionitis, neonatal death and handicap), and written consent must be obtained.

INDICATION

Any woman with relatively 'silent' cervical dilatation between 18 and 26 weeks – even women whose cervix is fully dilated – may be suitable. Some women may have some contractions which settle easily with gyceryl trinitrate (GTN) or other tocolytics. The cerclage should not be attempted until the woman has had at least 12 h without GTN and contractions have ceased.

Prior to inserting the suture the results of an up-to-date anomaly scan should be checked to confirm that the fetus is structurally normal. An amniocentesis may need to be performed, and the amniotic fluid should be sent for microscopy and culture, and the glucose level should be checked. Sufficient fluid may be removed to reduce the tension in the amniotic sac and aid insertion of the suture. The possibility of sending amniotic fluid for fetal karyotyping should be considered.

Chorioamnionitis, painful contractions, significant antepartum haemorrhage and ruptured membranes are exclusions to rescue cerclage.

Many women with 'silent' cervical dilatation will have a mucoid or slightly bloody show. The Amnistix may also test positive, even though the membranes are intact.

TECHNIQUE

Rescue cerclage should be discussed with the consultant and performed by personnel sufficiently skilled in the procedure. A classical or modified Shirodkar or MacDonald suture may be used. If the uterus is irritable following the procedure, the use of GTN should be considered. Prophylactic antibiotics in the form of erythromycin 500 mg four times a day and metronidazole 400 mg three times a day (one dose of each given preoperatively) and continued for 5 days should be considered.

If the woman ruptures her membranes, or shows any sign of chorioamnionitis, the suture should usually be removed immediately. Signs of early chorioamnionitis should be checked for (e.g. slight persistant pyrexia, abdominal tenderness).

The woman should be treated as being at high risk of premature delivery, and consideration should be given to the use of dexamethasone at 26 and 28–30 weeks. The suture should be removed electively at 36–37 weeks. A general anaesthetic should not be required, spinal or regional analgesia usually being sufficient.

BIBLIOGRAPHY

Edmonds DK, ed. *Dewhurst's Textbook of Obstetrics and Gynaecology for Postgraduates*, Sixth edition. Oxford: Blackwell Science, 1999:622
James DK, *et al. High Risk Pregnancy*. London: WB Saunders, 1994:1318

28

Female genital mutilation

INTRODUCTION

Preconceptual de-infibulation should be aimed for as the 'gold standard'. De-infibulation should be performed antenatally in pregnancy. However, if de-infibulation has not been performed antenatally, it can be performed in the first stage of labour

MANAGEMENT IN LABOUR

Discussion of the possible issues arising at the time of delivery should occur prior to labour, with the offer of examination to see the extent of the female genital mutilation (FGM). Involvement of interpreting and counselling services is often necessary.

POINTS TO NOTE

FGM constitutes a health risk to African women and can hinder the provision of appropriate obstetric/midwifery care. It is carried out sometime between birth and puberty. The degree of mutilation varies and clitoral damage is unpredictable. Classification of FGM is unhelpful and a poor indicator of damage. Each case of FGM needs to be assessed individually.

Use appropriate translators when needed (N.B. it is inappropriate to use a female translator who is in favour of FGM).

Very few women have the clitoris removed; it is usually buried under the scar tissue.

In some cases of infibulation the opening that is left may be only 0.5 cm diameter, and it may therefore take 15–20 min (or more) to empty the bladder.

TABLE 27-1. COMPLICATIONS OF FEMALE GENITAL MUTILATION

- Psychosexual problems
- Psychological problems (flash-back)
- Shock
- Haemorrhage
- Sepsis
- Mortality (1:10 according to the WHO)
- Problems with micturition
- Recurrent urinary tract infection
- End-stage renal failure
- Non-consummation
- Dyspareunia
- Infertility
- Vaginal infections

Management problems

Various issues are raised during the management of female genital mutilation:

- Diagnosis of urinary tract infections – it is difficult to obtain a 'clean' sample

- Diagnosis and treatment of infection

- Diagnosis and treatment of conditions such as ectopic pregnancy or fibroids because bi-manual examination is not possible.

- Problems of access during pregnancy and labour (e.g. it is often not possible to place a fetal scalp electrode)

FEMALE GENITAL MUTILATION INTACT (I.E. CLOSED) AND NOTED DURING THE ANTENATAL PERIOD

Reversal can mean that vaginal delivery is possible and may obviate the need for an extensive episiotomy (or episiotomies) at delivery. The optimum time for de-infibulation is thought to be 20 weeks (Personal communication, H. Gordon, African Well-Woman Clinic, Northwick Park Hospital, UK). Spinal anaesthesia is the anaesthesia of preference. It is best practice to avoid a reversal operation in labour for a known case of FGM.

IF FEMALE GENITAL MUTILATION IS ONLY NOTICED IN LABOUR

If FGM is noticed only in labour, the woman should be assessed by a senior specialist registrar or consultant. It is considered best practice to carry out a reversal in the first stage of labour

IF PREGNANT AND HAS HAD PREVIOUS VAGINAL DELIVERY

If a woman presents with FGM and has had a previous vaginal delivery, the state of the genital area should be assessed, paying special attention to whether she has been resutured after the previous delivery. There must be an adequate opening for vaginal delivery. If there is abnormal scarring, this can give way very suddenly and tear extensively, so must be investigated thoroughly.

SURGICAL REVERSAL

The aim of surgical reversal of FGM is restoration to normality. To ensure a greater chance of success, there needs to be:

- adequate anaesthesia, e.g. spinal for pregnant women
- an assessment of the scar (using a probe/dilator)
- an incision made in the midline to expose the urethra
- an extended incision (2–5 cm) to expose the clitoris, which is present in most cases

If the clitoris is damaged, it should be repaired using the clitoral stump. The labia should be repaired with 3/0 or 4/0 vicryl rapide. Re-suturing to the previous state is illegal and should always be refused.

POSTNATAL RE-EDUCATION

Women may need some re-education about what 'normal' micturition and menstruation will be like.

Community midwives need to pass knowledge of FGM to Health Visitors so that parental education can hopefully prevent FGM happening to female offspring of the family.

BIBLIOGRAPHY

Edmonds DH, ed. *Dewhurst's Textbook of Obstetrics and Gynaecology for Postgraduates*, Sixth edition. Oxford: Blackwell Science, 1999:622

29

Overwhelming sepsis

DIAGNOSIS

The classical features of sepsis are fever, vasodilatation, hypotension, tachycardia and tachypnoea. Patients may also show cyanosis, pallor, cold extremeties, hypothermia and jaundice. Labour ward staff should be aware of possible renal and lung involvement.

INVESTIGATIONS

Investigations used when evaluating a suspected case of sepsis are full blood count (white cell count raised, platelets lowered), clotting screen, urea and electrolytes, liver function tests, blood gases and/or pulse oximetry. Blood cultures and relevant samples should be taken for culture and sensitivity.

MANAGEMENT

When a case of sepsis is identified, the senior specialist obstetric and anaesthetic registrars should be informed. The patient should be moved to a high-dependancy room and given high-flow oxygen. A central venous line should be inserted and the patient should be given a colloid infusion.

An intensive care unit observation chart should be started and the patient kept on a strict fluid balance. Prophylactic heparin and antibiotics (blind) should be initiated, seeking advice from the on-call microbiologist.

Gentamycin 2–5 mg/kg/day should be administered in three divided doses (i.e. 80 mg intravenous three times a day). Labour ward staff should be aware of fetal ototoxic effects (withhold until after delivery if delivery imminent). In addition, intravenous (IV) metronidazole 500 mg four times a day and IV amoxycillin 500 mg four times a day should be administered.

Renal dose dopamine (2 µg/kg/min) should be considered to improve renal blood flow, and staff should always consider the transfer of the patient to the intensive care unit.

BIBLIOGRAPHY

Clements RV. *Safe Practice in Obstetrics and Gynaecology*. Edinburgh: Churchill Livingstone, 1994:492

Edmonds DK, ed. *Dewhurst's Textbook of Obstetrics and Gynaecology for Postgraduates*, Sixth edition. Oxford: Blackwell Science, 1999:622

James DK, et al. *High Risk Pregnancy*. London: WB Saunders, 1994:1318

30

Failed intubation drill

If intubation has failed, it will initially be necessary to ventilate the patient with 100% oxygen, maintaining cricoid pressure. Assistance should be called for.

If an airway is obtained and there is no urgent need to continue, the patient should be woken and a regional technique or awake intubation should be considered. If there is urgent need to continue, the airway (with oral or laryngeal mask airway [LMA]) should be optimized or intubation should be attempted again, continuing general anaesthesia.

If no airway is obtained, any of the following may be attempted:

- an oral airway
- release cricoid pressure
- LMA or
- cricothyroid access

31

Refusal to receive blood products or undergo medical intervention

REFUSAL TO RECEIVE BLOOD PRODUCTS

The absolute refusal to receive all blood products under any circumstances should have been clarified during the antenatal period by discussion with the relevant senior specialist registrar or consultant.

If this has not been done the specialist registrar or consultant on call should see the woman and discuss this issue. The result of the discussion should be recorded in detail in the notes. It should be clarified whether the woman would refuse all blood blood products if that was thought to be the only way to save her life. If this is so it should be recorded clearly in the notes.

CONDUCT OF LABOUR AFTER REFUSAL OF BLOOD PRODUCTS

After checking the mother's full blood count, the obstetric senior specialist registrar on call and the on-call anaesthetist should be informed. Labour in these circumstances requires active management of the third stage and postpartum syntocinon infusion.

If the haemoglobin level is below 10 g/dl, an intravenous line should be inserted when in labour to administer syntocinon 10 IU with the third stage and run a syntocinon infusion via a pump or giving set at 10 IU/h for 2 h. The on-call haematologist and on-call obstetric consultant should be informed.

The anaesthetic specialist registrar and obstetric consultant should be called early if there are any complications of labour involving haemorrhage.

REFUSAL TO UNDERGO MEDICAL INTERVENTION

If a woman refuses to undergo a medical intervention that the staff present feel is clearly indicated (e.g. Caesarean section) the the staff involved should call their immediate senior promptly (e.g. junior specialist registrar calls senior specialist registrar who should see the woman). If this process does not lead to a satisfactory outcome the obstetric consultant on call should immediately be informed.

BIBLIOGRAPHY

Clements RV. *Safe Practice in Obstetrics and Gynaecology*. Edinburgh: Churchill Livingstone, 1994:492

32

Sickle cell disease

INTRAPARTUM CARE

The stress of labour may precipitate a sickle cell crisis. The following guidelines should be followed in all women with sickle cell disease:

- Inform the Haematologist that the patient is in labour

- Encourage oral fluids (3 l/24 h)

- Continously monitor the oxygen saturation by pulse oximetry, and give oxygen by face mask if necessary

- Continuously monitor the baby

- If a painful crisis occurs treat as usual for that patient. Always seek a cause and always send a midstream urine (MSU) for urgent microscopy

- If strong opiates are needed notify the neonatologist and warn the patient that after delivery the baby may have to go to the special care neonatal unit

BLOOD TRANSFUSION

As a general rule patients with sickle cell disease should only be transfused because of a particular clinical situation, not just because they have sickle cell disease. Such situations might be their obstetric or haematological history, or clinical problems in a current pregnancy. The final decision on transfusion will normally be made together by the consultant obstetrician and haematologist. Possible indications include an ongoing high transfusion regime, multiple pregnancy, poor fetal growth or a haemoglobin 15% less than the steady state level.

Since any sickle haemoglobin in transfused blood will invalidate monitoring of the sickle haemoglobin percentage in these patients it is important that all blood for patients with sickle cell disease be screened for sickle haemoglobin (with the solubility test) prior to transfusion. Many patients with sickle cell disease require multiple transfusions and many of them already have red cell antibodies. It is, therefore, important they be screened for red cell antibodies prior to any transfusion and that appropriate blood be selected. The donor blood should be cytomegalovirus negative or, if this is not possible, leucocyte-depleted blood should be used. Since many of these develop significant iron overload, it is also important they have blood which is as fresh as possible (normally less than 7 days) when they are on a high transfusion regime so that the red cells last as long as possible.

For all these reasons it is essential that: a) the request form for transfusion be clearly marked indicating that the patient has sickle cell disease and b) that the transfusion laboratory be given as much notice as possible that a transfusion is required (often at least 3 working days) unless the transfusion is required as a medical emergency.

PUERPERIUM

Crises may occur in the puerperium, therefore watch infection sites (urine, caesarian section scar, intravenous line sites, perineum and breasts).

Good hydration should be maintained.

SICKLE CELL CRISIS IN PREGNANCY

Hospital admission to the obstetric unit, usually to the labour ward, is recommended for assessment and intervention. The haematology team must be notified promptly of the admission. Adequate analgesia must be given – diamorphine via a patient-controlled analgesia pump is usually effective.

The patient should be kept warm, well-hydrated and comfortable, while fetal movements should be checked and cardiotocography be performed. Full blood count (FBC) should be monitored and the patient should be screened for infection. Send an MSU in all cases. FBC should be checked daily if the clinical picture is not clearly improving.

BIBLIOGRAPHY

De Swiet M, ed. *Medical Disorders in Obstetric Practise*, 4th edn. Oxford: Blackwell Science, 1995:683

Edmonds DK, ed. *Dewhurst's Textbook of Obstetrics and Gynaecology for Postgraduates*, Sixth edition. Oxford: Blackwell Science, 1999:622

James DK, *et al. High Risk Pregnancy*. London: WB Saunders, 1994:1318

33

Peripartum collapse

CAUSES OR PERIPARTUM COLLAPSE

Possible features of peripartum collapse are numerous and are detailed below. Whatever the cause, two intravenous cannulae (16-G) should be inserted and oxygen should be given via a face mask, and the obstetric and anaesthetic specialist registrars should see the patient immediately.

Amniotic fluid embolism

Amniotic fluid metabolism is associated with multiparity and may precipitate labour, uterine stimulation and Caesarean section. It is characterized by sudden dyspnoea, fetal distress and hypotension followed within minutes by cardiorespiratory arrest and/or seizures.

Anaphylaxis

There may be cyanosis, hypotension, wheezing, pallor, prostration and tachycardia and/or urticaria.

Asthma

Asthma is characterized by wheezing and the use of accessory muscles for breathing.

Cerebrovascular accident
There may be a post history of headache suggestive of cerebrovascular abnormalities.

Eclampsia
Tonic clonic seizure associated with other features of pre-eclampsia.

Haemorrhage
Concealed abruption or uterine rupture are common haemorrhagic causes of peripartum collapse.

Myocardial infarction
Peripartum collapse can occur after a myocardial infarction and is sometimes seen in those with a history of heart disease with or without a current history of chest pain.

Tension pneumothorax
Sudden onset of pleuritic chest pain is suspicious of a tension pneumothorax. Diminished breath sounds are also present.

Pulmonary embolism
Apprehension, pleuritic chest pain, sudden dyspnoea, cough, haemoptysis and collapse are suggestive. An important differential diagnosis is pneumothorax.

Uterine inversion
Uterine inversion only occurs in the third stage. Profound hypotension is an important diagnostic pointer. Inversion maybe partial and therefore diagnosis not obvious.

AMNIOTIC FLUID EMBOLISM

In cases of amniotic fluid embolism, the obstetric and anaesthetic specialist registrars should be called. Cardiopulmonary resuscitation (CPR) should be initiated with high-flow oxygen and/or intermittent positive pressure ventilation (IPPV). At this point urgent delivery should be considered.

Two large-bore intravenous (IV) lines should be inserted and the patient infused with 2–4 units of Haemaccel until the blood pressure is normal, at which point the infusion should be stopped. Arterial blood gases, urea and electrolytes, liver function tests, full blood count and clotting should be checked and 6 units of blood crossmatched. Anaemia and/or coagulopathy should be corrected. The on-call haematology specialist registrar should be informed.

If uterine atony is present, it should be treated with syntocinon or carboprost (see Chapter 25). Hypotension may be due to cardiogenic shock and should be treated accordingly.

ANAPHYLAXIS

As soon as anaphylaxis is discovered, high-flow oxygen should be initiated. A large bore IV cannula should be inserted and 500–1000 ml of colloid should be infused rapidly to re-expand the intravascular compartment. Cardiopulmonary resuscitation or intubation for IPPV should be considered if necessary.

Adrenaline should be administered as 5 ml 1:10 000 slow IV, or via an endotracheal tube.

If wheeze is predominant, a salbutamol nebulizer should be set up to administer 2.5 mg in 2.5 ml of normal saline. Give hydrocortisone 100–200 mg IV over 2 min and chlorpheniramine 10 mg (i.e. 1 ml) IV over 1 min in all severe cases.

UTERINE INVERSION

If uterine inversion can easily be reduced it should be done manually, starting treatment for shock with IV fluids. If the placenta is attached and easily removable, it should be removed once shock is corrected.

O'Sullivan's hydrostatic reduction should be used if manual reduction is unsuccessful. The inverted uterus is held within the vagina by the operator and the introitus sealed with one or two hands of an assistant. Two litres of warm saline are infused into the vagina rapidly.

Once corrected, syntometrine 1 ml IM stat should be administered and a syntocinon infusion at 10 IU/h syntocinon via a syringe pump or giving set should be set up.

If this fails, the consultant on call should be informed and a vaginal or abdominal surgical approach should be considered with division of the cervix.

UTERINE RUPTURE

In cases of uterine rupture, an IV infusion should be set up, and haemoglobin and clotting studies should be performed. Six units of blood should be crossmatched. Immediate laparotomy should be performed under general anaesthesia. The senior specialist registrar must be present, and the consultant must be informed.

BIBLIOGRAPHY

De Swiet M, ed. *Medical Disorders in Obstetric Practise*, 4th edn. Oxford: Blackwell Science, 1995:683

Edmonds DK, ed. *Dewhurst's Textbook of Obstetrics and Gynaecology for Postgraduates*, Sixth edition. Oxford: Blackwell Science, 1999:622

James DK, *et al. High Risk Pregnancy*. London: WB Saunders, 1994:1318

34

Elective delivery of the fetus affected by severe red cell sensitization (e.g. Rhesus diseases)

In women who are undergoing elective Caesarean section for fetal rhesus disease the following must be done:

Two days before the intended day of delivery, two units of cross-matched blood should be requested, labelling the specimen "For neonatal exchange transfusion. Contact the paediatric neonatal specialist registrar if any difficulty with cross-matching". Write the date and time of delivery on the form.

On the day before delivery, the obstetric senior house officer (SHO) should check that blood is available for fetal transfusion.

On the day of delivery, the neonatology SHO should check that blood is available for fetal transfusion.

After delivery, the midwife supervising the delivery should take cord blood in order to establish bilirubin levels. It is essential that the neontal unit staff are aware of any delivery of a baby affected by rhesus disease and are present at the delivery.

Appendix I

The King's College Hospital protocol for closure of the labour ward and maternity beds

This policy has been formulated to ensure that, in the rare event that closure of the maternity unit is required, it can be managed in a consistent manner, with clear, safe, and planned alternative arrangements for mothers and babies. Closure would only be considered when all other potential solutions have been exhausted.

Closure has to be considered as part of the Trust Risk Management Strategy. It is the responsibility of the Midwifery Manager on call to implement the policy following discussion with the Director of Midwifery and the Consultant Obstetrician on call.

PROCEDURE TO FOLLOW FOR TAKING A DECISION TO CLOSE THE LABOUR WARD

General principles

It is critical to ensure that a safe standard of care can be provided for women and babies on the labour ward. This need may mean that, despite the fact that women have booked to have their baby at King's, the occasion may arise when it is safer for them to be diverted to another hospital.

It is important to recognise, however, that such action may, in itself, carry a risk which must be taken into account when the risk of the in-house situation is considered. Risks of diversion include:

- the time delay involved

- the fact that staff at the receiving hospital will not know the woman

- the anxiety caused to the woman and her partner

Wherever possible an impending crisis should be anticipated, and it is the responsibility of the Midwifery Manager on call, in co-operation with other senior midwives and the midwives in charge of the clinical areas, to review the bed and staffing situation on a daily basis, anticipate likely problems and to try to resolve them sooner rather than later.

SITUATIONS WHICH MIGHT LEAD TO EMERGENCY CLOSURE

- Staff absence resulting in inadequate numbers or inexperienced skill mix to manage high-dependency workload
- Insufficient bed availability on labour, ante/postnatal wards and no possibility of using beds in other areas of the Trust (to ascertain this contact should be made with the Clinical Site Manager)
- Shortage of midwifery or medical staff due to sickness/absence
- The outbreak of infection in clinical areas. (Again reference should be made to the Clinical Site Manager to ascertain bed availability in Trust)
- A major power failure or major incident

ACTION TO BE TAKEN BY MIDWIFERY MANAGER IF CLOSURE PROPOSED

Discuss the situation with the Director of Midwifery, review the anticipated workload against the midwifery establishment for the next 12–24 h.

Call the Obstetric and Paediatric Consultant on call. The decision to close the unit must be multidisciplinary.

The Midwifery Manager will inform the labour ward co-ordinator of the decision to close.

Prior to the closure arrangements the Midwifery Manager must ensure another maternity units will accept any labouring women and their babies. Once agreement has been obtained from a receiving unit the midwifery manager will contact the labour ward co-ordinator and ambulance control requesting diversion to the accepting maternity unit and inform the accident and emergency department. The anticipated time span for closure should be agreed and faxed through to Ambulance Control.

The Midwifery Manager will record the decision in the labour ward admissions book. Labouring women will be informed of the need for diversion as they telephone or enter the unit. Staff must ensure that women are made aware that they should take their notes with them.

REVERSING THE PROCESS

As soon as the precipitating factors have resolved and there are adequate facilities and staff, the reverse process applies. Inform the Labour Ward Co-ordinator, the Clinical Site Manager, the Accident and Emergency Department, the Obstetric and Paediatric Consultants and Director of Midwifery that the unit will be opening. Contact the receiving unit and thank them for their co-operation. Obtain details of any women who have been cared for so that we can write to them. Phone Ambulance Control and notify them of the unit reopening. The Director of Midwifery will write to any women who have delivered elsewhere.

Appendix II

The King's College Hospital guidelines for communication between midwives, junior doctors and consultants in relation to care of a woman in labour

1. INTRODUCTION

1.1. The Confidential Enquiry into Stillbirths and Deaths in Infancy (CESDI) and the Confidential Enquiry into Maternal Deaths regularly highlight the importance of midwives and doctors making appropriate referral of women in labour to more experienced staff when abnormalities occur.

1.2. The 1998 UKCC Midwives Rules and Code of Practice state under rule 40, "In an emergency, or where a deviation from the norm which is outside her current sphere of practice becomes apparent in the mother or baby during the antenatal, intranatal or postnatal periods, a practising midwife shall call a registered medical practitioner or other qualified health professional who might reasonably be expected to have the requisite skills and experience to assist her". This rule is applicable to all labour ward midwives.

1.3. The RCOG/RCM Report, Towards Safer Childbirth – Minimum Standards for the Organisation of Labour Wards (Feb 1999) states that:

"Full cover or Supervisory cover is applicable to units delivering more than 4,000 babies per year and/or tertiary referrals".

Just over 4000 babies a year are delivered in King's including tertiary referrals.

Supervisory cover is available defined as:

Forty hours of set consultant sessions on the labour ward, 40 h or 10 fixed sessions per week Monday–Friday. The consultant's work plan will indicate no other commitment during the labour ward session.

Out-of-hours on-call (18:00–08:00 hours and at weekends). The consultant must be available for the labour ward within 30 min. At weekends a daily labour ward round and either a physical or telephone round in the evening is required. The number of rounds will increase commensurate with workload.

1.4. King's is a teaching hospital and midwives and doctors are trained on the labour ward. It is important that a balance be achieved between the important service provision at consultant level for high-risk cases and the training of junior doctors and midwives in decision making.

2. LEVELS OF COVER

2.1. Obstetric
A consultant obstetrician, a specialist registrar year 4 to 5, a specialist registrar year 1 to 3 and a senior house officer (SHO) are rostered to cover the labour ward 24 h/day as documented on the monthly obstetric staff rota.

2.2. Paediatric
A consultant paediatrician, a specialist registrar year 4 to 5, a specialist registrar year 2 to 3 and an SHO are rostered to cover labour ward 24 h/day.

2.3. Anaesthetic
A consultant anaesthetist is rostered for five full days per week on the labour ward with no other clinical responsibilities. This consultant is supported by an SHO or specialist registrar. At night, cover is provided by a specialist registrar with no other clinical responsibilities. This doctor is covered by a senior specialist registrar on site and a consultant at home.

2.4. Midwifery
A midwifery co-ordinator for the labour ward is identified for each shift.

A supervisor of midwives is identified for every 24-h period and is on site 08:00–17:00 and on call 17:00–08:00.

A midwifery manager is identified for every 24-h period and is on site 08:00–17:00 and on call 17:00–08:00.

3. HOW TO CONTACT STAFF

3.1. Rotas for obstetric, anaesthetic and paediatric staff are kept on the notice board in the labour ward office.

3.2. The list of supervisors/managers on call is in the day-off duty book.

3.3. There is a communication board beside the main telephone on the work station on the labour ward. This has contact numbers (message pager, mobile telephone and home telephone) for all senior staff including obstetric consultants, specialist registrars, the lead anaesthetic consultant, midwifery managers and also for the community and practice midwives.

3.4. Each morning the names of the obstetric staff on duty are written on the communication board. Whenever staff change this is updated.

3.5. Outside the obstetric theatres, by the telephones, there is an information sheet showing the names, grades and pager numbers or bleep numbers of all the obstetricians, paediatricians and anaesthetists.

4. MIDWIFERY REFERRALS

4.1. All midwives caring for women booked under King's maternity unit for home or hospital births are required to adhere to the labour ward guidelines. Should any care given deviate from such guidelines the reason for this should be carefully documented.

4.2. The 1998 UKCC Midwives Rules and Code of Practice apply to all midwives working on the labour ward (see 1.5).

4.3. Each woman present on the labour ward is noted on the board in the labour ward office. This board also identifies the midwife allocated to care for that woman. The board is updated as soon as care is handed over to another midwife.

4.4. A qualified midwife can take full responsibility for the care of a mother in normal labour. However, when working on the labour ward at King's, all midwives must also ensure the co-ordinator is aware of the progress in labour of any woman for whom they are caring. This does not detract from an individual midwife's responsibility for the care but ensures good communication and a co-ordinated approach to running the labour ward.

4.5. The co-ordinator is also available to give support and guidance to midwives who may be less experienced than herself in looking after women in normal labour.

4.6. In the rare situation where the labour ward co-ordinator disagrees with the care given by another midwife to a woman in normal labour the supervisor of midwives on call should be contacted.

4.7. If a midwife decides to transfer a woman into hospital from a home birth she must contact the senior specialist registrar or consultant on duty who should advise the labour ward co-ordinator that a woman is on her way into hospital.

4.8. If a midwife is looking after a woman whose labour is high risk obstetric staff must be involved. Obstetric staff are responsible for planning the care of that woman.

4.9. If a midwife is looking after a woman in normal labour and an abnormality develops the obstetric team must be called. The labour ward co-ordinator or the midwife responsible for the case may do this, but in the latter situation the labour ward co-ordinator must be advised as soon as possible what is happening. This is to ensure good communication and a co-ordinated approach to running the labour ward.

4.10. A midwife transferring a woman in from a home birth with an abnormality in labour must refer that woman to the senior obstetric specialist registrar on arrival on the unit.

4.11. The midwife or the labour ward co-ordinator must, at all times, consider the appropriate level of referral. The person contacted must have the ability to deal with the problem. If a midwife is unhappy with the care proposed or the advice given by a member of the obstetric team she must contact a midwife with more experience or her supervisor.

5. REFERRALS BETWEEN THE OBSTETRIC TEAM

5.1. A senior specialist registrar or consultant must be present for all vaginal breech deliveries, all vaginal twin deliveries and all trials of instrumental deliveries in theatre.

5.2. In these cases (5.1) it should be agreed at the relevant labour ward round who will be contacted. The decision will be made by the consultant and will be principally dependant on the experience of the specialist registrar. The decision must be documented in the notes.

5.3. A senior specialist registrar must discuss the final decision for all emergency Caesarean sections with the consultant on call and would normally be present when this decision was made, particularly if the case was not known to him/her.

5.4. In any situation where the labour ward is extremely busy the consultant on call should be informed and the threshold for them taking responsibility for high-risk deliveries lowered. This will ensure the senior specialist registrar is available to support junior staff.

5.5. Although the consultant on call is responsible for all decisions during their duty span it may be appropriate for the senior specialist registrar to speak to the named consultant for that woman's care i.e. the consultant with whom the woman is booked. This would normally be discussed with the consultant on call. This may be because of a prospective request by the named consultant to be consulted or it may be because the woman is diabetic, is having twins, has psychiatric disease, etc.

5.6. If the consultant is to be off-site during the daytime at any time then that consultant should arrange cover by another consultant. The labour ward, senior specialist registrar and switchboard must be informed of this. If this is prearranged leave then the alteration should appear on the rota.

6. WARD ROUNDS

6.1. Good care planning and regular ward rounds during the working day can greatly reduce crisis situations emerging at night and improve team-work.

6.2. On weekdays, there is an 08:30 consultant ward round (09:00 on Fridays) and 13:00 ward review attended by the team of junior medical staff on call, the anaesthetic team and the labour ward co-ordinator. A consultant review also takes place at 17:00. This will be particularly necessary when there is a problem case or cases and when the specialist registrars have changed in the middle of the day. There will always be at least a consultant telephone review at 22:00. The senior specialist registrar will always phone the consultant unless there has already been recent contact. At weekends and on Bank Holidays there will be a consultant ward round at 09:00 and then further contacts by telephone or in person at regular intervals.

6.3. Junior medical staff conduct ward rounds at:
    Weekdays: 08:30, 13:00, 17:00, 22:00
    Weekends: 09:00, 13:00, 17:00, 22:00

Appendix III

Guidelines for termination of pregnancy following diagnosis of fetal abnormality or intrauterine death in the second trimester

REGIMEN FOR TERMINATION USING MISOPROSTOL AT KING'S COLLEGE HOSPITAL

1. Following requests for termination of pregnancy up to 30 weeks' gestation after diagnosis of major fetal abnormality or intrauterine death written consent should be obtained from the parents. A blue form must be completed in cases of termination of pregnancy.

2. Mifepristone (RU 486) 200 mg should be prescribed and given to the patient who should be observed for an hour after the medication.

3. Arrangements should be made for the patient to return at approximately 36–48 h after the mifepristone. On return, 800 μg (4 × 200 μg tablets of misoprostol) should be inserted into the posterior vaginal fornix. Liberal analgesia and an antiemetic should be prescribed, and an anxiolytic if wished.

4. Thereafter, 400 μg of misoprostol is given orally at 3-h intervals (maximum four oral doses). In the rare cases that the oral route may not be tolerated, misoprostol may be given vaginally or rectally. Abortion may not occur until the course is completed. No further misoprostol should be administered for a period of 12 h after these four oral doses. If abortion has not occurred within 24 h of starting the course, further management should be discussed with the consultant.

5. Delivery may be precipitate, especially in multiparous patients, after the first oral dose of misoprostol. The fetus and placenta may be delivered together. Occasionally there is delay between delivery of the fetus and the placenta. If further misoprostol is due during that interim period, it should be administered. As long as there is no excessive bleeding, the patient may be observed for up to 4 h following delivery of the fetus. If, after this time the placenta has not passed, speculum examination would be performed, as the placenta may be lying in the upper vagina. If this is not the case, evacuation under general anaesthesia may be required.

6. The patient should be observed for a period of 4 h following passage of the placenta before discharge home. If the bleeding becomes excessive at any stage, the specialist registrar should be informed.

Index

Printed and bound by CPI Group (UK) Ltd, Croydon, CR0 4YY

23/10/2024

01777674-0004